A Doctor's Eat-Hearty Guide for Good Health and Long Life

RICHARD G. MARGOLESE, M.D.
in association with
Harriet Margolese
and Jacqueline Margolese

Parker Publishing Company, Inc.
West Nyack, New York

© 1974 *by*

PARKER PUBLISHING COMPANY, INC.

West Nyack, New York

*To our families,
for whom it was done and
without whom it couldn't have been done.*

Library of Congress Cataloging in Publication Data

Margolese, Richard G
   A doctor's eat-hearty guide for good health and long
life.

   1. Low-cholesterol diet. 2. Heart--Diseases--
Prevention. I. Title. [DNLM: 1. Diet--Popular works.
2. Heart diseases--Prevention and control--Popular
works. WG113 M329d 1974]
RM237.75.M37   613.2'8   74-778
ISBN 0-13-216374-8

Printed in the United States of America

Foreword

It is a pleasure for me to write this short preface to an imaginative and possibly life-prolonging cookbook. I do it on two accounts: First, professionally, as a cardiologist interested in preventive medicine and, second, as an amateur gourmet. The most sophisticated tastes will be satisfied by many of the delicious recipes so clearly described in the pages that follow.

We are witnessing a raging epidemic of arteriosclerotic heart disease in most of the "civilized" world. The medical profession does not yet fully understand all the mechanisms resulting in heart attacks and their interaction. Despite ongoing, intensive, world-wide research, the answer to coronary heart disease still eludes us. However, as emphasized by Dr. Margolese, we *have* identified several "risk factors" that appear to be implicated when populations with a high incidence of heart disease are studied closely. As a result of such epidemiologic studies on the continent, in Europe, Asia, and Africa, there is widespread, almost universal agreement that, if we were to (1) modify our eating habits, (2) effectively control elevated blood pressures, (3) eliminate cigarette smoking, (4) maintain ideal weight, (5) remain physically fit, and (6) find a measure of equanimity in our lives, we would, no doubt, reduce the death and disability rates from this dread disease.

This book makes it easy to reduce the hazards of excessive saturated fats and cholesterol in our diet. Its philosophy is even more important than the actual recipes described. For, with adherence to the basic principles of a low-cholesterol diet described, the housewife, responsible for determining the nutrition of her family, will develop and become accustomed to a cooking and baking style that will be nutritious, delicious, and, hopefully, antiarteriosclerotic.

While all segments of the population can only benefit from a reasonable adherence to the dietary regimen elaborated by the authors, I especially recommend it to those persons who are a high risk by virtue of having abnormal blood fats, detected in appropriate analyses by their physicians, or who already have some evidence of coronary artery or other arterial disease, or whose family history includes close relatives with premature arteriosclerotic heart disease. However, I want to emphasize that dietary control alone, without regard to the other risk factors mentioned above, will not be enough. When you sit down to enjoy one of the many tasty dishes to be found in these pages, relax, don't overeat, and make mealtime a pleasant interlude in your daily life. Plan your schedule so it is possible to get some regular physical exercise, like walking briskly each day. Kick the cigarette habit if you have it (your food will taste so much better if you do), and see your doctor regularly. If you follow the Margolese approach in your cooking and eating, chances are your blood fats, if initially abnormal, will look a lot better in several months. Bon appetit!

Isadore Rosenfeld, M.D., F.R.C.P.(C)
Clinical Associate Professor of Medicine
New York Hospital—Cornell Medical Center

Introduction

American families are facing a serious and growing health crisis! Heart disease is our number-one killer and what is most alarming is that young men and women are becoming the victims of this disease with increasing frequency.

We have evidence that this disease begins in school-age children and progresses continuously and relentlessly. It is now apparent that not only the overworked, overstressed businessman is likely to have a heart attack. Rather, it is the average person—factory worker, clerk, or executive—whose life is in danger.

Why Me?

Heart attacks often occur without warning and can be fatal even in a person who appears to be in good health. You must understand that it is you, not some stranger, who is in danger. More important, you must also realize that something can be done about this threat—something simple, straightforward, and highly effective.

The Real Problem

At one time in North America, nutritional problems meant deficiency diseases. Today, many problems are caused by an *overabundance,* not a deficiency. We eat too much fat, particularly too much saturated fat. This book will clearly explain how improper eating plays a key role in the development of heart disease.

Scientific evidence on the causes of heart disease is increasing every day and includes a wide range of experiments and observations. In general, scientists find atherosclerosis and heart disease in countries with the highest standards of living where people eat too much cholesterol and fat, especially in the form of eggs, butter, whole milk, and meat. Our country certainly fits this description.

The American Heart Association has recommended the reduction of fat, especially saturated fat, in our diet as one means of preventing heart attacks. While other factors are also involved, diet control is presently the most practical way to protect your life from the high risk of heart disease.

What Does Diet Change Mean to You?

This is the key question, and its answer explains why this book will be particularly useful and special for you. Whether you are one of those who eat to live or live to eat, it is important to be able to enjoy your food. You will be reassured to know that you don't have to give up food you like to make the changes necessary to avoid the high risk of heart attacks.

Successful Method

This method succeeds because it is painless and simple. People can improve their food habits without feeling that they are missing anything they love to eat. Our plan allows you to enjoy taste treats you would be surprised to find in a health diet. The secret is basically a matter of substitution and the effort is minimal.

We provide no tables of cholesterol ratings or fat contents. There are no mathematical computations or conversions to make. All of this has already been done for you, so that you will automatically attain the proper shift in fat intake. Our book reads like any other cookbook —just cook as you always do, but follow our recipes and suggestions. The recipes provide dishes that have had their basic ingredients modified to make them more healthful than usual fare. You never feel you are eating "diet" food.

An important factor is that these changes can be accomplished *by anyone, using ordinary food available in the typical grocery store.*

How to Do It

In the first section of this book we have taken care to explain how and why the heart disease threat came into being and what you can do to remove this threat to your life. The second section tells how to implement our plan and the third section contains the recipes. Each recipe chapter opens with a small section explaining why certain suggestions or substitutions are made. This background is included in order to help you understand more clearly what you are doing when you follow our recipes. Ultimately, you will be able to proceed on your own, with full confidence and understanding.

Useful information on eating out and buying and preparing food is discussed. You will also learn how to avoid being fooled by the manufacturers and processors through knowledgeable label reading. In following this plan you will probably find that your family will eat a broader range of more interesting food than they ever did before.

Other Factors

The effect of cigarettes and what you can do to stop smoking are discussed in practical terms. A special chapter is devoted to the problems of being overweight. The secret of successful dieting is revealed and many of the fad diets are discussed and laid to rest. This is all vital information for anyone interested in sensible plans for better health.

Save Your Money

It is interesting to note that foods highest in fat content are often the most expensive items in the grocery basket. By following our methods of home substitution for so-called "convenience foods," you will find significant savings on your grocery bill. For example, home-made chocolate chips are about one-third the cost of the commercial type, which are also much higher in fat. Compare the cost of a cup of oil at 21 cents to a cup of butter at 38 cents. By this one substitution you save your money and your heart. Why not do more?

In summary, this book will convince you that heart disease is a real problem for *you*. It will show you why this problem exists and teach you how to deal successfully with it. The result will be good, hearty eating with the heart in mind.

ACKNOWLEDGMENTS

Thanks are due to many friends who helped so graciously in the work on this book. Special mention, however, should go to Eunice Palayew for her invaluable help in editing, Rose Mindel for helping with the compilation of the index, Harriet Lazare and Ronney Caplan for testing and proofreading, and Rhoda Tafler for her typing.

Acknowledgment is due Arlene Greenberg, Librarian at the Lady Davis Institute for Medical Research at the Jewish General Hospital, for her aid in research of the medical literature.

Thanks are expressed to *The American Journal of Medicine, The Journal of the American Medical Association,* and *The Journal of Preventive Medicine,* for kind permission to refer to scientific articles and statistics published.

And special acknowledgment goes to Ellen and Joel Margolese and their grandfather David Margolese for testing all the recipes, especially the ones that didn't make it into the final edition.

Contents

Chapter 1 · How Heart Disease Kills Without Warning

At the start of the 1972 baseball season, a popular hero, the forty-eight-year-old manager of a major league baseball club, died suddenly of a heart attack. Shortly before that a young swimming champion died suddenly from heart disease. You may remember that a twenty-seven-year-old member of the Honor Guard at President Kennedy's funeral died a few months after that sad event from coronary heart disease. Sudden deaths of young people attract a brief burst of attention, then are forgotten.

If you think about it for a minute, you will realize that you probably know someone who died recently of a heart attack. The fact is that each year 600,000 Americans die from coronary heart disease, making heart disease the number-one killer in America. Another 200,000 people die annually from diseases of the arteries, such as strokes, that affect other parts of the body. This is more than one American death from these diseases every minute, night and day.

Heart disease is not merely the number-one cause of death in our country; it kills more people than cancer and automobile accidents combined. This killer strikes all classes and age groups but, in recent years, there has been a relentless trend toward heart disease in young people. The average age of heart attack victims is steadily dropping.

Interestingly enough, while heart disease is the most common cause of death in our society, it is not so in most other parts of the world. Why should this problem be growing at such a dramatic rate in America? What are the factors that contribute to the phenomenal increase in heart disease deaths in our society? The answers to these questions are complex, but there seems to be at least one constant element that occupies a central role in discussions, in scientific study, and in government-supported research. This element is *fat*, and here we are talking not of the fat on your body, although that is important, but of the fat consumed in your diet.

Teen-age Heart Disease

To understand the role of fat, we have to go back to the early 1950s when authorities were shocked to see extensive evidence of heart disease in young, athletic people. It had always been believed that heart disease was part of the aging process, that it was unavoidable, and that only older people were affected. This complacent attitude was shattered forever in the 1950s. At that time autopsies performed on young American soldiers killed in the Korean War revealed a dramatic incidence of arterial disease. This shocking finding became even more significant when it was found that Koreans in the same age group, killed at the same time, did not show evidence of this disease. Neither group of soldiers died of heart disease; they died battlefield deaths; but the autopsies on the American soldiers showed a type of arterial disease that we know leads to heart attacks. This disease, called atherosclerosis, is characterized by the narrowing of blood vessels, which then leads to heart attacks.

The autopsy findings taught scientists an important lesson. They realized that this disease began very early in life, and that any eventual heart attack was only the end point of a long process. The importance of this turning point in scientific understanding should not be underestimated. Doctors were shocked to find that *a person who dies at age fifty or sixty from a heart attack actually began that disease process when he or she was a teenager.* That means that all of us, you and I, may unknowingly be furthering the development of heart disease in our own bodies, without realizing that anything is happening.

The fact is that heart disease does begin early. It strikes without warning and can be fatal to a young and unsuspecting person. Therefore, we all have good reason to find out what we can do to avoid becoming one of these shocking statistics. Our efforts at preventing heart disease must be directed to the basic questions of original causes, including the role of diet. It is the purpose of this book to go deeper into this problem and its answers.

Young Children

Even more astonishing than the Korean War autopsies were the results of later studies prompted by these battlefield findings. One of these was an analysis of autopsies done on young American children, aged six to ten, who died in traffic accidents. The unexpected results revealed that atherosclerosis was beginning even earlier in life than had previously been suspected. Comparison of results with some other countries confirmed these findings of heart disease appearing at early ages. However, there were large areas of the world where this disease did not occur in young people.

These paradoxical findings sparked extensive discussions among scientists and public health authorities to find the explanation for these discoveries about our society's health. Many reasons were entertained and explored, but one interesting factor has emerged and continues to be important in these discussions. *This factor is diet.*

Our "Good" Life

Countries with living standards and diets similar to those in America seem to have the same incidence of heart diseases. But other countries, such as Japan or China, have a significantly lower incidence of these diseases. It is interesting to note that these countries differ from ours in that their staple protein food is not meat; large amounts of grain-based foods are eaten instead of large amounts of animal fat. We will return to this important difference in a later chapter.

Eating Habits Play a Role

In our country we can make an interesting comparison with our relatives or ancestors who lived in other countries. There is often a difference in heart disease incidence, and this seems to relate to diet more than to genetic makeup. For example, Mediterranean people, such as Italians or Greeks, living in North America and eating an American diet, have the same incidence of heart disease as other ethnic groups of Americans. However, there are a few small towns, settled long ago by groups of immigrants, where assimilation into the American culture has not taken place. These people continue to live on diets very much like those in their native land. In these situations, interestingly enough, the incidence of heart disease is as low as in the home country. This is a fascinating indication that the food people eat is an important factor in the development of heart disease. Those people who adopted North American eating habits also adopted an increasing incidence of heart disease.

The same results were found when the situation on the other side of the continent was examined. Japanese and Chinese people who eat an American diet have a significant number of heart attacks, but those who eat like their Asian counterparts do not.

Another startling example of how food habits can affect health is found in Norway. Here, the land and the people can be divided into two general groups. There is a steep, rocky seashore bordered by high mountains that separate the coastal regions from fertile valleys in the interior. The rocky seashore supports fishermen, and the mountains, until recent times, kept them fairly well isolated from the rich, inner valleys that feature cattle-grazing lands. This geographical division leads to two types of natural diets: fish and oils predominate in the coastal regions; meat and dairy products in the interior. The statistical results from this division are just what we would expect. There is a higher incidence of coronary disease in the central regions where the people eat meat and dairy products and a lower incidence in the fish-eating coastal areas. These naturally occurring differences in diet and heart disease have pointed the way for our investigation.

The next step is to perform scientific studies in which people are fed a controlled diet containing a specific amount of fat in order to see the effect of the fat on the development of heart disease. These studies have been done and more specific illustrations of the role of fat as a cause of heart disease will be given in later chapters. But the few preceding examples of the association of heart disease with diet provide very good epidemiological evidence for diet as a causative factor.

Epidemic

The term "epidemiological" derives from Greek words meaning "upon people." This is a fancy word that public health authorities use, but I am introducing it here to underscore an important point. An "epidemic" does not have to be a contagious disease. When a disease increases alarmingly in a specific population due to a basic underlying factor or factors, it may be termed an epidemic. Many authoritative scientists have referred to our national heart disease problem as an epidemic. It is important to realize, whatever word or phrase is used, that a serious health problem exists. This means that the next victim could be you or a member of your family—your husband, wife, or child.

There is often no way to tell where you stand. People who have just had complete medical checkups, with normal electrocardiograms, have suffered heart attacks. It is important, therefore, to find out what you can do to reduce your chances of having a heart attack.

Small fragments of evidence are relentlessly building the case for the need to reorganize our national dietary habits. Fortunately, there is much that we can do as individuals to accomplish meaningful changes and this is the reason for the extensive recipe section of this book. The next few chapters will explain more about this problem and give you some of the answers.

Chapter 2 • What You Should Know About Your Heart to Enjoy a Long and Healthy Life

Mr. K., a busy accountant, would listen to his doctor explain that he had already developed some heart disease and would have to modify his diet. At each visit, he admitted following the diet for a week or two before losing interest and returning to his regular diet that contained too much fat. At these repeated checkups there was no evidence that his progressing heart disease was under control. His doctor soon realized that because his patient did not understand exactly what was happening to his heart and blood vessels, he was not sufficiently motivated to diet successfully.

At last his doctor explained in simple words how the heart works so that Mr. K. could clearly see the relationship between the diet he had to follow and his heart disease. With this understanding, he now had the proper motivation to maintain his diet, and both he and his doctor are satisfied that the effort has been worthwhile.

We will, therefore, now look at what happens in heart disease. To understand this, we must first look at the heart to learn what it is and what it does.

Actually, the heart is little more than a simple physical pump. It has none of the biochemical sophistication of other organs such as the kidneys or the liver, and has no job to do except pump blood.

The flow of blood, therefore, is the essential element in our discussions. The first primitive animals on earth consisted of only one cell and needed no heart because they derived their nutrition by direct absorption from the sea water that surrounded them. In the same way, all the cells of a human body derive their nutrition from the modern equivalent of sea water—blood. When single-celled animals, such as the amoeba, began to evolve into complex multicelled animals, such as the human, they had to develop a circulatory system to keep their "sea water" bathing all their cells. This is the reason for our circulatory system, and this is why our blood is still salty like sea water. Anything, therefore, that interferes with the flow of blood through the blood vessels really interferes with the life process itself. And the presence of a disease that interferes with the normal flow of blood means that the life of the cells being supplied is in jeopardy.

Blood Flow—Energy and Life

Everything we do requires energy. The basic use of energy is simply moving our muscles in order to breathe, but the work of digesting and the work of thinking also require energy. Moving our muscles and moving ourselves around similarly requires energy. The energy comes from the food we eat; just as an automobile engine burns gasoline to produce energy to move the car, so do our cells burn sugar from the food we eat to produce energy. The sugar, then, is our fuel. Just as the gasoline engine produces exhaust fumes, the body produces exhaust chemicals, such as carbon dioxide, that must be carried away from the cells by the blood. It is carried to the lungs where the exhaust gases are exchanged for fresh oxygen, and the cycle is repeated with every heartbeat and every breath. Many complex chemical reactions go on in our cells to do the things just described, and they all depend on the flow of blood pumped by the heart.

Your Body's Rusty Plumbing

The disease called atherosclerosis involves the production of small irregular deposits, or rough spots, on the smooth, inner lining of the blood vessels. These are deposits of a fatty substance called cholesterol, which soon become surrounded by an inflammatory reaction and scar tissue; the whole complex process is called "atherosclerotic plaque." As this disease process continues, these "plaques" enlarge and occupy more and more of the inside of the blood vessel. Just as rust can build up in a plumbing system in a house and cut the flow of water to a trickle, so too can these plaques build up in the arteries and cut the flow of blood to a trickle. If the flow of blood diminishes too far, the lives of the cells being supplied are in danger. If the flow stops, these cells will die. It is particularly alarming to realize that the flow can diminish to a very dangerous point while causing no symptoms or cardiogram signs. That is why so many people have sudden heart attacks with no previous warning that anything is wrong.

Your Heart's Simple "Pump"

The heart has a muscle that is actually built into its wall; this muscle does the pumping. Like any other muscle, the heart requires its own supply of fuel and oxygen and requires continual washing with blood to carry away the waste products, such as carbon dioxide. For this purpose, the heart requires its own blood supply; it cannot obtain sugar and oxygen from the blood it pumps through itself to other organs. Therefore, the muscle of the heart has its own blood vessels to serve these needs. See Illustration 2-1 for your blood traffic flow.

Causes of Heart "Pump" Failure

The arteries supplying blood to the heart muscle are called "coronary arteries." If they don't supply it with enough blood, the heart will weaken, producing heart failure. If any of these arteries are blocked, the heart cannot do its pumping work and may even stop. This is what happens in a coronary thrombosis or heart attack. "Thrombosis" means blockage of the artery by clot; this happens when a plaque becomes so large as to narrow the artery to the point where blood flow is so difficult that it clots and flow stops.

While many of our vital organs come in pairs, such as the kidneys and the lungs, we have only one heart with no spare to depend on. The whole heart process depends on the health of the coronary arteries. *Even a professional football player, in perfect physical condition, depends on these two small arteries for life!*

The same disease process can affect other arteries in the body and indirectly affect the heart. If other arteries become diseased, they also become narrow and lose their elasticity. Since the heart has to pump blood through all these diseased vessels, it will have to work harder by pumping more forcibly and more frequently to provide the same amount of blood to the rest of the body. It is not surprising to learn that the heart that works harder against more resistance will fail sooner. This, indeed, is what often happens.

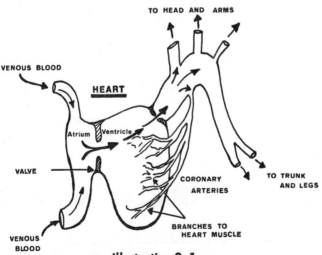

Illustration 2–1
Your Blood's Traffic Pattern Pumped by Your Heart

Strokes—A Similar Problem

When the atherosclerotic process occurs in the brain, it will cause a narrowing and, therefore, a lessened blood supply to part of the brain. If a large blood vessel is blocked, the result will be a major stroke. Loss of smaller blood vessels produces so-called unnoticed minor strokes, often associated with changes in personality. A series of minor strokes occurring over a period of years is what we believe produces senility.

The same process, atherosclerosis, can occur in the eyes, producing poor vision and blindness, or in the legs, causing gangrene, which may lead to amputation.

In order to understand this discussion better, it is necessary to define some phrases that are becoming commonplace.

Coronary arteries:
Those blood vessels that supply the muscle of the heart with blood for its own nutrition.

Coronary thrombosis:
The presence of a blood clot within a coronary artery producing complete blockage of flow to that section of the heart.

Myocardial Infarction:
The technical term for the death of part of the heart muscle; almost always caused by coronary thrombosis.

Atherosclerosis:
The process of buildup of fibrous tissue and cholesterol in the lining of blood vessels producing a rough area or plaque that continues to grow and forms the base for a blood clot eventually blocking the artery.

Arteriosclerosis:
A word similar to atherosclerosis meaning virtually the same thing.

Angina or Angina Pectoris:
Chest pain, usually caused by narrowing of a vessel to the point where blood flow is inadequate, but not to the point where the heart is permanently damaged. This often occurs during a period of exertion, when the need for blood rises, but the ability of coronary arteries to deliver blood is limited. The pain forces the patient to stop the exertion, allowing the heart to relax and the pain to subside.

We have seen that serious diseases result from the type of blood vessel narrowing called atherosclerosis. We have discussed briefly the role that fats play in causing this disease. At this point it is necessary to examine more carefully the exact role that fats and food play in the actual development of blood vessel and heart diseases.

Chapter 3 • How Does Heart Disease Happen?

There are actually many causes of atherosclerosis and the degree to which the disease develops depends on many factors. Think of how a traffic jam depends on many factors such as weather, road repairs, time of day, or a stalled car. Some, or all of these factors must be present in just exactly the right combination to produce the expected result. For example, at four o'clock in the morning, you wouldn't expect a real traffic tie-up even if all the other factors were present.

The development of a disease like atherosclerosis is similarly dependent on many factors, in a very specific combination, having a specific result. Some of the elements involved are natural resistance, family history, diabetes, high blood pressure, stress, and obesity. An exact combination of some or all of these will produce a heart attack in a given patient. It is this requisite for exactly the correct combination that explains why one or another of the individual factors does not always produce the attack by itself. Natural resistance, for example, explains why not everyone working in the same office gets a cold when one member of the group has one. Natural resistance must be one of the factors in such a disease as atherosclerosis. However, even natural resistance cannot be relied upon if the other elements are present in strong enough form. Everyone should consider himself a possible target for heart disease.

We can identify many of the specific factors associated with atherosclerosis, and evaluate them as we would evaluate a traffic jam.

Actually, atherosclerosis affects just about everybody to some degree. But in some people it can be more severe and progress more rapidly because of the effects of many factors that are associated with the development of atherosclerosis.

Family History

There are certain situations in which family history seems significant. Although everybody has some degree of atherosclerosis, some families have more, and these families also have a higher rate of heart disease and coronary failures. Since one cannot choose his parents, other factors causing atherosclerosis must be considered and eliminated if found.

Blood Pressure

The presence of high blood pressure is another factor associated with an increased incidence of heart attacks. There is little dispute among medical authorities about the need to control high blood pressure; this is something that can usually be accomplished with proper medication. Although there are many causes, the presence of high blood pressure may often be an indication of narrowed blood vessels due to atherosclerosis.

If many of the body's blood vessels are narrowed, the heart must pump harder against this high resistance and the blood pressure goes up. High blood pressure means that the heart is working harder to force blood through the blood vessels to the organs and tissues that need it. Therefore, whatever the cause, blood pressure should be controlled as much as possible by medical treatment in order to minimize the continuing strain on the heart.

Diabetes

The presence of diabetes seems to be correlated to some extent with the development of strokes and heart attacks. Doctors in most hospitals routinely screen their patients for the presence of diabetes and recommend early treatment in an attempt to minimize the effects of the atherosclerotic process and the other effects of diabetes.

Smoking

Arterial diseases are significantly higher in smokers than in non-smokers, and giving up smoking will clearly lessen the risk of these diseases. Virtually the entire medical profession has agreed on this. There is no magical way to give up smoking; those smokers who have a great deal of difficulty need medical advice or guidance on how to do it. By one means or another, they must find and exert the will-power necessary to quit for good. (Chapter 6 gives more information about this.)

Diet

Most of the just-mentioned factors can be controlled or modified to slightly lessen the chances for arterial disease. The role of diet rates special mention because, with the possible exception of blood pressure control, diet is the most manageable factor associated with coronary artery disease. The benefits of successful management may be greater than for any of the other factors. In many ways managing the diet is simpler to do than giving up smoking—ask any smoker who has tried to quit—not that the smoking factor should be ignored. There are many reasons why it is felt that diet is implicated in this disease process, and a more careful analysis of these factors is now in order.

We know that the process called atherosclerosis can be caused in animals by feeding them a diet high in cholesterol and fat. As early as 1913, a Russian scientist reported that rabbits on a high-cholesterol and high-fat diet developed this arterial disease. Abundant evidence has been gathered in the years since then connecting dietary problems to the development of arterial disease.

We have also learned that people who live luxuriously on a diet rich in all nutrients have a high degree of atherosclerosis, while people on substandard diets, low in calories and animal fats, are relatively free of the disease. When the cholesterol level in the blood is measured, it is found to be higher in the more affluent group. Thus, there is a relationship between diet, cholesterol in the blood, and heart disease. This relationship has been studied intensively to find out which element is primary and produces the others.

Heart Disease Is a Disease of the Affluent

Actually, three-quarters of the world's population eats the more primitive, less nourishing diet, but most of their fat intake is in the form of fish or oil. The United Nations statistics for the postwar era show that the United States and Canada consume 135 grams of fat per person daily. It is only during recent years that North Americans have been eating this increasing proportion of fat and cholesterol; this is reflected in the rising incidence of heart disease. It is a clear fact that our diet has improved in the twentieth century in vitamin and mineral content; we do not often see deficiency diseases such as scurvy and rickets. It is paradoxical that during this same time span our increased fat intake has become detrimental to our health. We are less healthy today, in this respect, than in the past.

Many animal experiments have been conducted to shed more light on this problem. The overwhelming majority revealed that when a variety of experimental animals were fed diets very rich in fats, they rapidly developed the atherosclerotic changes that we see in humans. These animal studies led to a closer look at human arterial disease.

What Large-scale Surveys Showed

The best way to study a disease process in humans is to select a large group of people called a "study population," and observe them for signs of the disease in question as well as for all the other variable factors that may play a role in the development of that disease. By observing societies and their regional eating habits, it would soon become apparent whether the suspicion of dietary origins of heart disease were justified.

Several large public health studies were undertaken, such as the famous Framingham study in Massachusetts. This was a large-scale evaluation of a whole community. Copious data were collected about the living and eating habits of the subjects. Many far-ranging factors such as age, sex, occupation, stress, and physical characteristics were measured. The investigators confirmed that increased levels of cholesterol in the blood were directly correlated with increased risk of coronary artery disease. They found that of all the different blood tests available to predict heart disease, blood cholesterol measurement was the best indicator, and that dietary fat intake was an important factor in the development of heart disease.

Effect of Fat on Human Survival

Another important group study of the role of diet was carried out in New York City. One hundred young men who had suffered a previous coronary thrombosis were placed on a low-fat diet and were compared with a second group of men, matched for age, occupation, type of heart disease, and so forth. The second group maintained their normal diet. The two groups were therefore identical, except for the different amount of fat in the food they ate. The second group had a 160 percent higher rate of recurrent heart attacks and a 233 percent higher mortality rate over the next five years compared to the group on the special diet.

Looking at these results another way, we can see that a person could double his chances of survival simply by changing his diet, since none of the other factors were altered. This is very strong statistical evidence in favor of diet change as a means of trying to diminish the chance of suffering a fatal heart attack.

Further Proof

Another important study, undertaken by the Veterans Administration Hospital in Los Angeles, has shown that some heart attacks and brain strokes could be prevented by diet control. The experiment done in that hospital compared two groups of people, randomly selected, to follow a normal diet or a specially modified low-fat diet. Chance alone decided which group a person was placed in. With enough people in the study this meant that all other factors such as age or family history would be equalized between the two groups.

Equal numbers of people were in each group; however, there were forty-eight heart attacks or strokes in the special diet group and seventy in the normal diet group. There was also an obvious reduction in blood cholesterol level among the people receiving the special diet, showing once again that by changing your diet, you can lower your blood cholesterol and lessen your chance of having a heart attack.

A study performed in Finland involved two mental hospitals. This is a suitable way to conduct such an experiment because it involves a rather stable population of people under stable conditions. In other words, because they are hospitalized people, the daily routine, life, stress, and habits are very much the same for both groups throughout the length of the experiment. In one hospital the regular diet was administered, and in the other, a special diet, modified for low fat was served. Serum cholesterol became much lower in the experimental hospital than in the normal or control hospital, and the rate of heart disease in the experimental hospital was less than half of that for the normal food hospital. After six years of steady, predictable results, it was decided to exchange the diets between the hospitals, so that the control hospital became the experimental hospital and vice versa. All other factors were left unchanged. In a short while, cholesterol level and cardiogram results reversed between the two, indicating that diet alone was the significant factor responsible for these changes.

The Effects of Fatty Foods

These surveys have studied the disease results in groups of people with diets that contain very specific fat content. Food normally contains three basic elements: carbohydrates, proteins, and fats—some amount of each element is always present. If the amount of fat is increased in a diet, then the amount of the others is usually decreased proportionately. When we speak of proportions we often talk of percentages. For example, a diet may be described as 30 percent fat, 30 percent carbohydrate, and 40 percent protein. In our country it is the increased amount of fat in general, and of one type of fat in particular, that seems to be the crux of the problem.

It seems, then, that diets that contain less fat have a significant effect in minimizing the risk of coronary artery disease; the reverse is also true. *Over the entire world, populations with diets high in fat have a high incidence of blood vessel diseases.* The only exception to this seems to be people whose diets contain fat in its oil state, such as among Arctic peoples who eat a great deal of seal and whale oil and fish products. This provides an important clue about specific kinds of fats that must be further explored.

The Two Main Groups of Fats

There are two main groups of fats—saturated fats and unsaturated fats. The difference between them is explained in the following chapters, but the essential point is that they have opposite effects on your heart and arteries. Saturated fats are harmful and unsaturated fats, such as the Arctic people eat, are healthful.

In the scientific experiments described so far, we have talked about diets low in fat. To be more specific, these diets were low in saturated fat. We shall see how, on an average diet, the saturated or unhealthy type of fat increased; this is our prime concern.

Why Do We Eat So Much Fat?

We know historically that human beings did not eat much fat until modern times. Modern conveniences such as refrigeration and improved transportation methods have meant easy distribution of fat-containing foods to our cities and our populace in ever-increasing volume. Prior to these developments of civilization, fats could not be consumed far away from the places where they were produced, nor could they be stored for long periods of time because they spoil. On the other hand, because cereals and other grains do not spoil, they have been the basic food staple throughout most of human history, and still are in many countries today.

Our food habits during the past thirty years have become increasingly harmful, leaning more and more toward commercial food processing and storage, both of which require an increased amount of saturated fat.

Dairy herds have been increased in size and have been specially bred for higher butterfat content in their milk. Similarly, animals bred for slaughter have been developed for "desirable" aspects in their meat, such as fat content and "marbling" in the red meat.

Many unsaturated oils, which are basically not disease producing, have been treated to provide properties considered better from the commercial point of view. Changing these into shortenings and margarines that are more convenient to use and keep better than the original oils also changes them into saturated fat, which causes the diseases previously discussed.

Scientific Proof of the Deadly Effects of Saturated Fat Foods

Scientists often like to double check, or prove their theories, by examining them from the opposite or negative point of view. If saturated fats in the diet produce heart disease, then the absence of fats in the diet ought to have the opposite effect. If this can be shown to be true, it would help to prove that saturated fats are instrumental in the development of heart disease.

This type of proof is available. During World War II, the affluent dairy-producing countries of northern Europe and Scandinavia were deprived of their normal diet by the occupying German forces that commandeered most dairy and meat products. However, the people were able to survive on available levels of grain and protein. Several studies conducted later by their governments and the United Nations confirmed that during these periods and shortly thereafter there was a significant decrease in the incidence of coronary artery disease among these populations—in spite of the greatly increased stress due to the Nazi occupation. After the return of peace and normal eating habits, the incidence of heart disease rose once again, and it has continued to rise. Since then, there has been other evidence that atherosclerosis is reversible—the first sign of reversibility is the disappearance of fat and cholesterol from the microscopic deposits on the inner lining of the blood vessels.

What Do These Studies Mean to Us?

These convincing studies and group experiments are very important pieces of evidence. What makes them all the more relevant are the confirmations we see when we look at individual people who bear out the expected results. The case of a forty-eight-year-old office worker is a good example. Mr. L. had never felt better in his life when he had a sudden heart attack. Although he made a good recovery, he continued to feel depressed and unhappy. After discussion, it was apparent that his depression stemmed from a feeling of dismay over his vulnerability to heart attack. He wondered if he could ever get back to a useful way of life.

To ease his mind, it was only necessary to provide him with some background information about heart disease and give him instructions about how to diet. With this renewed sense of purpose and the feeling that there was something concrete he could do to help himself, he went on the diet enthusiastically. A recent checkup years after his heart attack showed that his cholesterol level had become normal and that there were no further signs of trouble.

Effects of Fats on Young People

In chapter 1 we learned that autopsies on young children who were victims of automobile accidents revealed the beginning signs of heart disease that would show up in later life. In order to check this further, the Department of Nutrition at Harvard University's School for Public Health did a diet study on adolescents in nearby prep schools. Students were divided into groups and given different diets. The results fit the clearly developing pattern, showing that more fat means more heart disease.

This was an important study, not only because it confirmed the idea that diet and cholesterol levels had a provable relationship early in life, but because it was possible to show that young people, who are not motivated to diet for reasons of possible future heart disease, can successfully lower the cholesterol content in their blood by following a special diet provided for them. *The secret is that the special diet was indistinguishable from their normal diet*—French toast made without butter, whipped cream without fat, cheese without 60 percent of its harmful fat, all the cookies and cakes they could eat with no worry about unwanted butter or shortening.

The Protection This Book Gives You

The recipes and instruction sections of this book do just the same for you. Anyone will now be able to provide himself with the same kind of protection provided by the Harvard researchers and we will show you how.

It is now over half a century since it was first shown that cholesterol and fat in the diet would lead to the development of atherosclerosis. Repeated studies such as those discussed in this chapter have shown that people with high levels of cholesterol in their blood have an increased risk of heart disease, and that diets high in cholesterol and saturated fat tend to raise blood cholesterol levels, while those low in these substances tend to lower blood cholesterol levels.

One important fact learned during the past fifty years is that there are different kinds of fat. Implications of the importance of these various types of fat and their relationship to heart disease are revealed by such peoples as the Eskimos, whose high-fat diet has not promoted atherosclerosis. Something inherent in the fat itself must account for the difference between the way high-fat diets affect Eskimos and the way they affect Americans. A chemical difference in fats is this factor. In the next chapter we will investigate the varying characteristics of fats to learn how we may profit through improved dietary management.

Chapter 4 • How Fats "Sneak Attack" Your Heart

As the scientific world plunged deeper into the investigation of fats, diet, and heart disease, it became clear that it was worthwhile to divide fats into two or three main groups, considering their effects separately. Fats are actually an essential part of everyone's diet, but you can have too much of even a good thing, and too much fat is especially dangerous. There are several types of fat, but the danger actually comes from eating too much of one of these types.

To understand the difference between the types of fat, it is helpful to reduce chemical complexities to simple examples. To do this, let us think of fat as a freight train. (See Illustration 4-1.) There are long chains of carbon atoms coupled together to make a fat molecule, like freight cars coupled together to make a complete train.

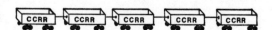

Illustration 4–1
Basic Structure of Fats Resemble a Freight Train

These atoms may or may not be chemically combined with hydrogen, and this difference is crucial. We can depict the combination with hydrogen as a freight car loaded with material. When the long train has all the hydrogen it can hold, it is called saturated. (See Illustration 4-2.)

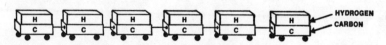

Illustration 4–2
Saturated Fat Train

Each carbon atom can hold two hydrogens by chemical "bonding." The molecule is conveniently depicted as in Figure 4-3, but this is obviously the same thing as the "freight car" illustration.

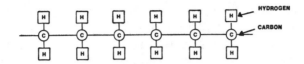

Illustration 4–3
Saturated Fat Molecule

When any hydrogen atoms are missing, the molecule is called *unsaturated,* and can then accept or react with hydrogen or other elements. (See Illustration 4-4.) Another way of expressing this is to

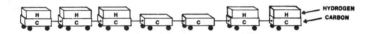

Illustration 4–4
Unsaturated Fat Train

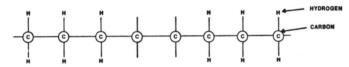

Illustration 4–5
Unsaturated Fat Molecule

say that saturated fats are chemically stable, because all the carbons are saturated with hydrogen and therefore cannot easily combine with other elements.

An unsaturated fat is one in which there are available bonds to react with hydrogen, or with other chemicals, to produce a different substance. An example of such a reaction occurs in certain oils, detected by an odor indicating that the oil has become rancid. The tendency to become rancid is a common property of unsaturated fats, caused by their chemical instability. This means that foods made from unsaturated fats will spoil more quickly. An unsaturated fat can be converted into a saturated one in order to prevent or delay this development. This is done by adding hydrogen to make it chemically inactive and stable. Food processors will frequently do this to "improve" their product.

Saturated fats are otherwise obtained from animal sources and are referred to as "animal fats." They occur naturally in butterfat products such as milk, cream, cheese, and butter, and in the meat of cows, sheep, pigs, and so on. This fat is solid at room temperature; the molecule is stable and doesn't react or change very easily.

Unsaturated fats are usually derived from grains and tend to be liquid at room temperature—for example, safflower, corn, cottonseed, and soybean oils. The main exception to this is *coconut oil, which is highly saturated.*

Food Industry Forces Changes on Us

Unsaturated fats are often called essential fats because they seem to be necessary for life and health. There is increasing evidence that diets containing larger amounts of these unsaturated fats will help prevent coronary artery disease. Unfortunately, these fats are becoming less common in our diet, and the saturated fats, which are associated with increased incidence of arterial disease, are becoming more common. One of the main reasons is the tendency of unsaturated fat to become more rancid. This means that the shelf and storage life of a product containing unsaturated fat is shorter, which is economically undesirable for the food-producing industry. From the processor's point of view, it is better to convert these fats into saturated forms for commercial usefulness. The result for the consumer is more saturated fat and less unsaturated fat in our food.

Hydrogenated Fats and Oils

The process of converting an unsaturated (or desirable fat) to a saturated fat (or undesirable fat) is called *hydrogenation*. Hydrogenated oils then, are those that are treated chemically to increase their stability and give them the solid properties required for shortening and margarine, i.e., the conversion from oil to a semisolid or solid.

The list of ingredients on many grocery products will often indicate the presence of "hydrogenated vegetable oils." Many modern products such as vegetable shortening began as unsaturated fats, and have been converted for industrial reasons.

With modern food processing, packaging, and patterns of consumption, man is creating his own disease situation. Our present habit of buying precooked food means we are consuming ever-increasing amounts of food that have been modified. We do not know the contents of all these products, but we would if they were cooked at home. However, we do know that for commercial reasons there is a relentless increase in the use of saturated fats and coconut oil.

The same holds true for food served in restaurants. A good example of this is seen in the small individual packages of "cream" served with coffee. Many of these are actually not cream, but vegetable oil, treated chemically to become saturated. These substitutions are worse than the cream itself from the point of view of saturated fat and health.

The Cholesterol Factor in Heart Health

An important part of this discussion is cholesterol itself. Cholesterol is a complex molecule and it, too, is essential to life in certain quantities. However, it seems to be detrimental to health when it is consumed in the excessive quantities found in the average American diet.

Cholesterol is present in all animal products, but is highest in egg yolks, shellfish, and organ meat such as liver, pancreas, and brain. Cholesterol is the basic building block with which the body makes many hormones essential to life. However, more than the minimal amount of cholesterol that one needs is obtained with any reasonable food intake, and most people in North America consume far in excess of this level.

Cholesterol Derived from Fat

Fats in the diet affect blood cholesterol levels, even when the level of cholesterol intake is unchanged. Saturated fats in our food tend to raise the blood cholesterol level because the body can make cholesterol from these fats. Thus, without consuming any extra cholesterol, your blood level will rise if your diet contains too much saturated fat.

Fortunately, certain unsaturated fats have the reverse effect. These can be divided into two subgroups—polyunsaturated, which means many open chemical bonds and monounsaturated, meaning one open bond. (See preceding illustrations.)

Eating more polyunsaturated dietary fat tends to reduce the blood cholesterol level, even when you eat the same amount of cholesterol.

Monounsaturated fats appear to be neutral in their effect on cholesterol and on the development of atherosclerosis. These fats are generally found in some vegetable oils such as olive oil.

Experiments indicate that saturated fats are twice as effective in raising the serum cholesterol as unsaturated fats are in reducing it. In other words, just as in weight-reduction dieting, it is far easier to be bad than good. Many saturated fats are added to our food during processing and preparation, thereby invisibly raising our consumption of these fats. For example, shortening and egg yolks are in cakes and cookies, and account for a large proportion of the saturated fats that we consume. Products such as snacks or crackers also contain these fats. Convenience foods such as snack meats, canned stews, and frozen dinners are all high in fat. Even lean-looking meat contains a significant amount of fat running between the muscle bundles. This is invisible to the naked eye, but some can be seen in the drippings when the meat is cooked.

Most cheese on the market contains large amounts of saturated fat, and people consume fair quantities of these cheeses. All this suggests that, without knowing it, we are eating too much saturated fat and not enough unsaturated fat. (How to deal with this problem is discussed in more detail in the sections called Grocery Shopping and Menu Planning.)

Deficiency Disease

One interesting way of looking at the problem is to consider that most Americans suffer from a deficiency disease. The highly unsaturated fats that are beneficial to health are being abandoned by industrial food processors and we are getting less and less of these essential fats in our food. In other words, changes in food habits and food processing techniques have resulted in a deficiency of a common food element that we once had in proper amounts.

As in any deficiency disease, it is necessary to correct the problem by obtaining proper amounts of the essential ingredients. The solution, however, lies not just in the absolute amount of unsaturated fat, but rather in the proportion of unsaturated to saturated fat.

Protection Against Cholesterol Effects

It is just as important to decrease the saturated fat as it is to increase the unsaturated. Thus, protection against coronary artery disease will result if we:

—increase unsaturated fat content
—decrease saturated fat content
—decrease cholesterol itself

Because of the complexity and interdependence of these factors, it is not clear at present whether it is more significant to do one or the other. However, because of their interrelationship, it is virtually impossible to do one of these without somewhat affecting the others. We think it is wisest to attempt to change from saturated fat to unsaturated fat as much as possible, giving you the advantages of both approaches.

Food Habits to Be Reconsidered for Better Heart Health

It is clear that we all eat too much fat in the form of animal fat and that some reversal of our habits will be necessary. Because meat, which is protein, is unavoidably combined with animal fat, it appears that eating meat to obtain an adequate amount of protein will provide an excessively high and unhealthy level of fat. Protein without the unhealthy fat content can, however, be found in fish, poultry, and grains.

1798525

Effect of a Fatty Meal on Your Heart

While we have good statistical evidence that a diet rich in saturated fat will lead to higher blood cholesterol levels and higher incidence of heart attacks, scientists often require more direct evidence to link a suspected cause to a disease. This direct type of evidence is available.

It is possible to examine the actual flow of blood in certain experimental animals through a microscope. For example, there is a way to do this in the hamster. Under mild anesthesia, the cheek pouch of the hamster can be turned inside out without ill effect to the animal.

The cheek lining, a thin membrane showing the flow of blood, is examined under a microscope. Normally the blood flows through the membrane like traffic traveling along a busy highway at an even, normal pace. When the animal has been fed a diet of whipping cream in an amount equivalent to a normal fatty meal in a human, we see the effects on the flow of blood shortly afterwards. There is thickening and sludging; the flow slows down markedly in the smaller vessels; in some, it stops completely. Six or eight hours later, as the effects of the meal wear off, the smaller capillaries start to show blood movement again, and the vessels open gradually until the flow returns to normal. It is easy to imagine how permanent stoppage of blood can occur with a clot inside the blood vessel, and it is not hard to imagine what repeated episodes would bring.

As in all scientific experiments, it is important to know that the results were actually caused by the fatty meal itself, and not because of the unnatural, experimental treatment of the animal. Therefore, this same experiment was done on the same animals on other days. They were given the anesthetic and the same size meal, but with low fat, keeping the pouch exposed for the same length of time. This time we see no evidence of slowing or stoppage. The experiment was often done in reverse using a low-fat meal first, and the high-fat meal following, but always with the same results.

This experiment provides highly specific evidence that fat in a meal can affect the flow of blood. We previously learned that fat in the diet can cause progressive narrowing of the walls of the blood vessels. When these two observations are put together, it becomes easy to understand why heart attacks occur more frequently in people whose diets are rich in fats and cholesterol.

The Exact, but Simple, Diet Change to be Made to Help Save the Heart

Too much of our food is taken as fat and too much of our fat is taken in "saturated" form. Something must be changed, but what to do can be perplexing. Most family doctors themselves are not too clear in their own minds about what to do and what not to do.

One particular colleague instructed a patient, Mrs. S., to lower her saturated fat intake, but neglected to explain that she should also increase her unsaturated fat intake to compensate. This meant that she was consuming almost no fat at all. The result was that the diet was impossible to maintain because of its dryness. Even more important was the fact that the diet was lacking in oils (found in such things as salad dressing) that would have been beneficial because they lower cholesterol levels.

It was then suggested that she add these unsaturated fats to her diet. Her diet once more became palatable as well as healthy.

Summary of Fat and Cholesterol Effects on Your Heart

We now know conclusively that heart attacks are more likely to occur in people who have higher levels of cholesterol in their blood and that the level of cholesterol in the blood depends on many factors. As we have seen, this level depends mainly on the amount of cholesterol and the amount of saturated fat you eat. By decreasing either of these you will decrease your serum cholesterol level. Practical and palatable diets can be devised with such a low daily intake. You will have little difficulty providing you have an understanding of the objective and how to reach it by diet changes.

Chapter 5 • The "Fats" of Life for a Healthier, Stronger Heart

Despite all the accumulated evidence, there has been half a century of debate about whether or not widespread changes should occur in the American diet. Today, according to a report from the United States Department of Public Health, the debates should be concerned not with whether changes should occur, but how extensively to apply these changes in a population that is riddled with atherosclerosis. The government thinks this is important enough to commit ten million dollars in research.

Despite this, many family doctors remain unconvinced or are sufficiently uninformed about what should be done. Since this type of diet change could be adapted rather simply, it seems to boil down to a decision to do something that is prudent, but not particularly difficult or revolutionary. To put it as a straightforward question: *Why not follow a low-fat diet before the heart attack strikes?*

There are many cases where heart disease is unsuspected and there are no warning signs of an impending heart attack. There are also cases, however, where no heart attack has actually taken place, but microscopic damage to the heart occurs and progressive scarring slowly robs the heart of needed power. Take the case of Mr. N., a factory worker with a good job and teen-age children. His blood cholesterol was found to be above normal and although he never had a heart attack, moderate damage and scarring caused excessive fatigue, partly because the heart could not perform effectively with diminished blood supply. He went on a long-term program of fat control and lowered his cholesterol well into the normal range. After two years on the diet he feels better, gets more out of his job and family, and has had no progression of his cardiac abnormalities.

The Unexpected Heart Attack

At the other end of the spectrum are the cases of patients with no symptoms and no warning of any kind about heart trouble. This is the kind of patient who has a sudden, unexpected heart attack, even though he may have just been given a clean bill of health by his doctor. Heart disease is so widespread that either of these types can occur in anybody. Everyone has some degree of atherosclerosis, and sooner or later may become one of the victims we have been talking about. Everyone can expect to benefit from proper diet control, and many people could actually prevent a heart attack from happening.

Foods as Preventive Medicine

Changing some of the basic dietary elements might sound like a major and difficult undertaking. The truth of the matter is that with available methods of buying and preparing food, it can actually become quite simple.

What to Do?

In 1969, the World Health Organization of the United Nations concluded its official report as follows:

Coronary heart disease has reached enormous proportions, striking more and more younger subjects. It will result in the coming years in the greatest epidemic mankind has faced, unless we are able to reverse the trend by concentrated research into its causes and prevention.*

National statistics show that millions of Americans have already modified their diet. In New York City, there is an anticoronary club made up of young and middle-aged men from all walks of life who have a common interest in preventing heart disease. These men meet for a coordinated attack on the cause and prevention of heart attacks; they consult with their doctors for individual management, as well as for group experiments that the doctors manage. Under the direction of doctors in the Department of Nutrition of New York City, these men have altered their normal food intake and now eat the kind of food described in this book. Their replacement of butter and shortening by margarine and oil, and the shifting of other fats from saturated to unsaturated, have resulted in a remarkable lowering of the incidence of coronary artery disease, and thus they have reduced the rate of recurrent heart attacks in their group.

Necessity for Dietary Changes

These and other diet studies previously discussed have shown conclusively that dietary changes are necessary. But dietary changes

---

* World Health Organization, 1969 Official Report, United Nations.

require motivation and this can sometimes be a problem. For example, in one early experiment 41 percent of the subjects left the study because of the monotony of the food, the effort required to follow the diet, and their longing for the foods that were forbidden on their diet. We have devised ideas and recipes in this book to avoid just that kind of situation.

One housewife we know, Mrs. K., encountered great personal difficulty in trying to follow instructions for dietary change after her husband had had a heart attack. The need for dietary change and the role diet plays in controlling the progress of the disease had been explained to her. Her family, however, had always taken great interest and pleasure in their food—indeed, they were robust eaters. Although they realized they should cooperate for the sake of Mr. K., they were really quite disappointed in the resulting low-fat diet. The result was growing dissatisfaction and strong temptation to abandon the diet.

What they really wanted, it turned out, was the enjoyment they used to derive from their old foods. When Mrs. K. learned about our system of *substitutions* everything changed. She was able to make many of her favorite recipes and everyone returned to eating with gusto but with one important difference: Mr. K. was now getting all the protection his doctor prescribed and so was the rest of the family. Everyone was now satisfied.

It is important to minimize what could be negative feelings about a healthful diet by providing foods as close to the forbidden type as possible.

Why Fad Diets Fail

Most people in North America have had some experience with dieting, usually for weight reduction, and for most people these have been unsuccessful efforts. Generally these diets are *too restrictive,* and quickly *become monotonous* with their confined taste experience. Because of the limited range of food allowed by most weight-reducing diets, the craving for other foods becomes greater and greater. Finally, the reward of having lost a few pounds is accepted as satisfactory and the person quickly abandons the diet, returning to previous food habits. We can easily see why it is often unreasonable to expect someone to follow a strict diet for any length of time.

Another complicating factor is that usually only one person in the household is following a special diet, and forbidden goodies may be around to tempt him. Since it is clear that the dietary aspects of coronary heart disease start in early childhood, it seems that modifications should really take place for everyone in the household. In this way only one kind of cooking is required for all; no special meals are needed for the dieter. As a matter of fact, it is very important to teach children the "fats" of life as part of their early food learning habits. This makes it easier for them to adopt a proper attitude in later years.

The Case of Mrs. B.

Mrs. B. had a problem similar to Mrs. K., but tried to solve it in a different way. She cooked low-fat meals for her husband and regular meals for the rest of the family. Although Mr. B. accepted the restricted meals because he realized it was important, Mrs. B. soon became overwhelmed by the added work and strain of double cooking. But worse than that, Mr. B. soon found himself eating forbidden food again.

Imagine her relief, and her husband's pleasure, when they learned that low-fat cooking was beneficial to everyone in the family and could be easily extended to please them all. Mrs. B. cooked with a new enthusiasm and no longer felt guilty. Her husband not only ate a proper diet, but even ate foods he had not expected to find listed in his diet, especially since Mrs. B. was now planning meals with a freshly stimulated interest resulting from the new ideas opened up to her.

Sticking to an Eating Program

Clearly, only a regimen or eating program causing minimal disturbance for the household can be successful in the long run, and only simple procedures will be expected to work on a large scale. Anything too demanding or too complicated will soon be abandoned by most of the people involved; it is for this reason that the methods advocated in this book are made as simple and straightforward as possible.

It is important to understand this very basic concept of our plan —it is universal in its application. It is easier to cook this way for everybody than to cook the old way for some and a special way for the dieter. We have already shown you convincing evidence that even young people must diet to prevent future heart disease, but it will be difficult to keep these youthful eaters on a serious program if it means giving up foods they like.

The Case of Mrs. S.

Mrs. S. wanted to help her husband, the victim of a recent heart attack, but she felt guilty because she knew she was not following the suggested diet plan for her husband, and asked her doctor for further advice on how to accomplish this. Her main problem was that she felt she couldn't deprive her growing boys of the foods they liked and wanted, and yet she couldn't manage to serve two types of menus. The result was that she sacrificed more and more of the diet factors her husband required.

Once the problem was defined, the solution was easy. First, the need to include her boys, for their own sake, in the plan was made clear to her. But more important, she was shown how to accomplish this in such a way that they would think they were still eating a normal diet. Now she only prepares one set of meals—one that everyone can and should be eating. You can do the same thing for your family, using this book as the key to success in this venture.

How to Handle This Book's Eating Programs

You can choose anything in the book, prepare it according to the recipe given, and automatically eliminate a significant part of the saturated fat you might have eaten had you cooked in your old way. You can still plan meals much as you did before—chicken, meat, fish, cookies, cakes, pies—they are all here, even mousses and pastries, but they are all modified to save you from eating harmful fat. For example, instead of using shortening when making a pie crust, you can use oil. For the same amount of work, you will have a healthful pie crust and start on the road to proper eating.

If you follow our recipe plan for all your cooking, only you will really know that the cooking has changed. *Meals will look and taste the same*—only now they will be healthy, not fat-loaded and unhealthy.

How This Book's Program Can Help You

Rather than forbid a food or a dish, the wise method would be to attempt to replace it, or at least those ingredients that are harmful to your heart. Someday, safe commercial substitutions will probably be available, but today commercially prepared foods, because they are loaded with fat, are more dangerous than home-prepared foods could be. It is, therefore, up to the individual homemaker to provide the substitutions within the home. The basic point of our method is simply to replace some of the common food components, such as butter and shortening, with safer ingredients, such as oil. You will then be eating foods that are similar, but will not cause cholesterol levels to rise, producing the subsequent effects of coronary artery disease.

Thus it is possible to improve your health by changing your diet while continuing to enjoy your customary wide range of taste experiences. It will be necessary to deny yourself only a few, limited foods completely, while substituting some basic ingredients in many others to change them from harmful to healthy.

It is basically the work of the wife and mother to safeguard the members of her family against heart disease by providing healthful foods. Adoption of simple, but prudent habits for better future health begins with this step, but must gain the cooperation of the whole family to be totally successful.

Chapter 6 • How Smoking Damages Your Heart

There is no longer any reasonable doubt about the relationship of cigarettes to disease and death. It has been proved conclusively that cigarette smoking is a major cause of lung and bladder cancer as well as chronic lung diseases such as emphysema and bronchitis. Smoking is also strongly implicated as a major factor in heart disease and the risk is proportional to the number of cigarettes you smoke.

An average smoker who consumes one to two packs of cigarettes daily increases his chances of having a fatal heart attack by as much as five times that of a nonsmoker. We have already learned how prevalent heart disease is in our society due to many other factors that may not be avoidable. Remember that a smoker is not only subject to all of these factors, but he quintuples his risk by smoking.

How Does Cigarette Smoke Affect the Heart?

One of the main constituents of cigarette smoke is nicotine. Nicotine is a poison that ranks in toxicity with cyanide. Drop for drop, it is equally dangerous. *A single drop of pure nicotine on the human tongue would be fatal.* Fortunately for smokers, nicotine is not pure in tobacco smoke, but it is there, and it does have its effect. Its main effect is to narrow the arteries by causing the muscles in the walls of the arteries to constrict.

The arteries have circular muscles that can constrict to decrease the flow of blood through that point. This is a necessary and normal function to control the flow of blood to different organs. These muscles act as valves and, by constricting, can close down the artery so that less blood gets through. For example, when running, blood flow is allowed to go to the leg muscles by the narrowing of blood vessels to other areas and by the opening of the muscle controls on the arteries supplying the legs. Another example is the way the blood flow can be increased to the stomach and intestines when digesting food by narrowing the blood flow to the skeletal muscles during the after-dinner period of relaxation.

Normally, some arteries are open and some are closed, so that the heart pumps blood into the proper number of blood vessels. If all blood vessels are narrowed simultaneously by a drug such as nicotine, the effect is to increase the resistance against which the heart must pump the blood. The heart itself is one of those organs that must get blood; nicotine creates a situation where the heart needs more blood to do the extra work of pumping against a higher resistance and is actually getting less. When you think about this process it is not hard to understand why cigarettes are associated with an increased heart attack rate.

It is also important to consider what happens to the tissue at the other end of the artery. If the artery is narrowed, the flow of blood, even with the heart working extra hard, may be inadequate, resulting in a deficiency of blood and oxygen for the cells in that tissue. This lack of oxygen may be serious enough to do harm. For example, there is a specific disease of the blood vessels called Buerger's disease that causes a different type of narrowing than that seen in atherosclerosis. If a patient with this disease smokes, the extra narrowing caused by the nicotine, added to the narrowing already present, almost always leads to death of the cells in the toes and feet due to lack of oxygen. This is called gangrene and inevitably results in amputation of the leg.

One such patient, Mr. N., already had gangrene in one leg and seriously diminished pulses in the other when he was advised to stop smoking. Despite the entreaties of his doctors, he refused to give up cigarettes, and the result, within less than one year, was amputation of both his legs above the knee. Not everybody needs the same warning for a specific disease, but many are receiving the general message about cigarettes and many like Mr. N. are ignoring sound medical advice.

Other Poisons

In addition to nicotine, normal cigarette smoke contains arsenic, lead, carbon monoxide, and formaldehyde—the smoker is treating himself to all of these with every cigarette he smokes.

Experiments You Can Do to Discover for Yourself the Deadly Effects of Cigarettes

Pulse Test

Many people do not believe in the validity of these facts about cigarettes and often feel "it can't happen to me." There are several simple experiments that one can do to illustrate the truth of the information on cigarettes. One myth easily exploded is the concept that cigarettes relax you. Many people feel that they enjoy a cigarette after a good dinner and can unwind and relax better because they smoke. It is only necessary to sit down comfortably and have someone count your pulse for one minute. Now, light up a cigarette and smoke it; then repeat the pulse count. The result may surprise you! Have you ever heard of someone who relaxed by driving his heart faster?

This after-dinner cigarette, by the way, is also shifting blood away from the digestive organs, frustrating the body's normal mechanisms of digestion. It is also killing your senses of taste and smell, thereby diminishing the sensory enjoyment of the meal. I know many people who have told me how much better their food tasted after they had become nonsmokers.

The Handkerchief Test

Another fascinating experiment involves the use of a clean handkerchief held across the open mouth. While the smoker blows a mouthful of smoke he has not inhaled into his lungs through the handkerchief, the clean linen will be stained by a reddish-brown color caused by the tar in the smoke. The experiment should then be repeated, this time inhaling the smoke deeply into the lungs in a satisfying (to the smoker) way. This second stain will be much lighter in intensity. The difference in the colors represents the amount of tar that remained in the lungs when the cigarette smoke was inhaled. Just imagine the effect of repeating this dozens of times a day—you will then have a good idea of what a smoker's lungs look like.

Other Experimental Proof

Cigarette tar can be applied directly to the skin of a laboratory rat to see what its chemical effects will be. Interesting enough, after a few weeks, a cancerous tumor will appear at the site of application—not by injection, just by simple contact application. It is this same tar that a smoker is introducing to the far more delicate tissues of the lung passageways.

On a simple level, there is a more direct effect cigarettes have on every smoker. We know that the irritant effect of smoke on nasal and chest passages can cause cancers. But we also must remember the body's more common reaction to these irritants; there is a loss of normal defense mechanisms that leads to an increased rate of common colds, sore throats, and other simple infections. Smokers lose twice as much time per year from work (and play) as do nonsmokers.

The effects of air pollution are also much more severely felt in a smoker's lungs than on a nonsmoker. The paralysis of our air passage defense mechanisms by cigarette smoke means that nature's way of trapping and filtering out unwanted particles is lost. Thus, when we breathe midcity air, or walk into a smoke-filled room, it is only the nonsmoker who can deal with this efficiently. The smoker breathes it into the deep recesses of his lungs and adds the effects of these pollutants to those of the cigarettes he has been smoking.

The Relationship Between Smoking and Heart Disease

Even with the risks of lung cancer being as high as they are, it is probably the chance of a heart attack that is the most serious risk a smoker runs. The incidence of heart attacks in this country is alarmingly high to begin with, but it is five times higher for a smoker than for a nonsmoker. This is a significant difference and one that should convince any smoker to stop smoking—here and now.

Why It Is Difficult to Stop Smoking

One of the hardest things to do in life is for a smoker to stop smoking. However, one of the reasons it is so hard is because most people just do not believe that smoking is a threat to health. When the Surgeon-General of the United States makes his annual announcement about the risks of smoking and cites the number of people who die because they smoke, the impact on the individual is lost because it is perfectly normal to say "He can't mean me—I only smoke twelve cigarettes a day," or "But I don't even know anybody who has died from smoking." The truth is he does mean you—and you really do know people who have died because they smoked. They may have had cancer caused by cigarettes, and you may not have learned the exact diagnosis, but I am convinced that you do know such people. You can also be sure that some of those relatives, neighbors, or acquaintances who have died from heart attacks would not have died when they did were they not smokers. So it is important to realize that it can happen to you. This realization is the key to stopping.

I remember a particular friend who I tried to convince for a long time to stop smoking. When I finally said that I was very upset to see someone about whom I care very much doing such a dangerous thing as smoking, he stopped to think for a minute, and realized he had never really thought about it in personal terms. He resolved then to stop immediately, and has been completely successful to this day.

How to Stop Smoking

A reliable, consistent, simple way to stop smoking is among the most elusive of man's wishes. There are as many plans to stop smoking as there are people who want to stop. The fact that there are so many ways to stop indicates that no specific plan has won the acceptance of most people as the best or easiest way. The only conclusion is that there is no best way or simple way. People smoke for many different reasons and thus their motivation to stop differs, too.

For some, simply reading these facts will be enough to convince them of the need to stop, and they will. For others there will be internal debates and many decisions to stop "tomorrow." People have devised ingenious plans to thwart their own ability to obtain a cigarette; for example, placing all the cigarettes in the furnace room wrapped in a package that must be unwrapped deliberately before being able to get a cigarette. There are commercial aids to stop including a plastic cigarette to hold in your mouth—a pacifier! Other aids are a series of increasingly efficient filters that reduce the smoke ultimately to zero, nicotine-flavored chewing gum, and even hypnotism.

A Doctor's Advice on Stopping Smoking

The only advice I can give to the smoker is to think very seriously about the risks and dangers of smoking and to make up his mind in a cool, deliberate way to stop. He can then devise his own reasonable and workable plan. For some this may mean stopping abruptly and completely, for others it may be better to decrease according to a pattern, such as no smoking at home and increasing the abstinence until no smoking at all is achieved. It is often helpful to devise a reward system that need be little more than recognition of success by the family. Set up special dates such as one month without smoking, then six months, and so on. Perhaps a special meal or dessert for the successful nonsmoker could be arranged. It is surprising how powerful a force family encouragement and recognition can be to a person who is struggling by himself.

The important prerequisite, however, is to admit that cigarettes really are dangerous and to agree that it is very possible that *you* can become a victim.

What Do Cigarettes "Cost" You?

Because they lead to such a high incidence of disease, it should be obvious that cigarette smoking will shorten your life. You may have seen statistics claiming that each cigarette means so many minutes off your life. Actually, there is a more accurate way to look at the effect of smoking. You can't add eight minutes to your life by skipping your next cigarette—that is a meaningless number. But you can compare your chances of outliving a nonsmoker. For example, nearly everyone born since the 1940s will survive to age thirty-five; death due to disease is very rare in young people. But in middle years, things can begin to go wrong and just over 20 percent of the people who don't smoke will die before age sixty-five. However, among people who smoke heavily, 41 percent will be dead before age sixty-five. The death rate for moderate smokers lies in between. Your chance of dying young is nearly doubled if you smoke regularly. It doesn't matter whether it is lung cancer, bronchitis and emphysema, or heart disease. The simple fact is that cigarette smoking will cost the smoker something, in health, in years, and in dollars, and there is no way to avoid these payments.

Chapter 7 • Will I Lose Weight by Following the Menus in This Book?

Nothing has been said so far in this book about how much you should weigh. Whenever we have talked about fat, we have meant the kind you eat, not the kind that is on your body. It is now time to discuss this latter type of fat because it has its own role to play. There is no doubt that being overweight is one factor that increases your chance of having heart disease.

It is estimated that for every pound of fat on your body there are twenty miles of blood vessels through which the heart must pump blood. If you think that this makes the heart work harder, you are correct. However, you must also consider the additional factor of the added weight in physical terms. It means that *you* must work harder just to move across a room. Imagine a person whose ideal weight is 150 pounds, and who is twenty-one pounds overweight. This is the same as if the person weighed 150, and each morning he strapped on a knapsack weighing twenty-one pounds and carried it around with him all day. This additional work by the overweight person also means his heart must work harder, and anyone who is overweight is imposing this extra load on his heart. Therefore, the statistics that tell us that obesity is a serious factor in heart disease are understandable.

Statistical Proof That Being Overweight Will Decrease Your Life Expectancy

A look at the tables of the Metropolitan Life Insurance Company will show you that your chances of living to age seventy are seriously diminished if you are overweight. For example, someone who is fifty-one and is markedly overweight has a life expectancy of sixteen additional years, whereas another person of the same age and of normal weight can expect to live twenty-two years, or six years longer. That is a lot of time with your grandchildren that can be lost if you are lazy about something this important! Remember though, even if you bring your weight down, the amount of saturated fat that you eat is still important and still must be dealt with.

Why You Will Lose Weight with This Book's Menu Program

It is interesting to note that simply by following the low-saturated-fat diet explained in this book, you will probably lose weight *if you are overweight*. Weight loss results when you avoid foods rich in saturated fat, because you automatically lower the intake of total fats at the same time.

The total amount of fat you eat is important in weight control because fat is very high in calories, and its relationship to the proteins and carbohydrates you eat is crucial.

A Calorie Attack on Your Heart

The three main foodstuffs are called fats, carbohydrates, and proteins. Any food you eat belongs in one of these three groups. Eating one gram of carbohydrate or of protein will produce four calories for your body to deal with. However, eating one gram of fat will produce nine calories—more than twice as much. It is the total amount of calories that you eat and expend in a day that determines whether or not you will gain weight. You need fuel to run your body; the energy of this fuel is measured in calories. Any excess amount of calories over the energy you require will result in weight gain. Whether the excess is taken as carbohydrate, protein, or fat, the excessive calories can be converted by the body into fat that is stored for a future day when there may not be calories available.

We cannot store more than an insignificant amount of carbohydrate and, therefore, fat is nature's way of saving up for a rainy day. It just so happens that in our society, with our eating habits, we have very few rainy days, and because we are very good savers when it comes to this particular commodity, most of us find it easy to become overweight.

How to Lose Weight Healthfully for Your Heart's Sake

The number of diet plans that people have tried is probably as numerous as the number of overweight people. Every time you open a popular magazine or look at the drugstore paperback rack, you will see another such plan—diets based on grapefruit, cottage cheese, martinis, meat, protein, carbohydrate, or what have you. Logic alone will tell you that the reason there are so many different diet plans is that none has proven to be superior to the others. This doesn't mean that they don't work. As a matter of fact, they all work and this is why they fail. Although that sounds contradictory, closer analysis will explain.

Your body is accustomed to receiving a certain amount of fat, carbohydrate, and protein each day, and has become adjusted to this. From this intake, it can extract the energy it needs, and perhaps store up some for future use. If there is no excess, the books are balanced at the end of the day and your weight is stable. Any diet plan in which you eat only one or two basic foods in large quantities and avoid others leads to a drastic dislocation of your body metabolism. The body is shocked by the sudden withdrawal of one foodstuff and the presentation of an excess of another.

Inside the body fats, carbohydrates, and proteins are converted into each other, but this takes several days and it is during this time that you lose weight. The body is unprepared for the sudden diet change, and begins to mobilize its reserves in order to compensate for what it thinks is an inadequate intake. Therefore, it burns up some of the fat it has stored, and some weight is lost. But about the time the body has finally settled down in its adjusted phase, the dieter becomes disenchanted with the diet because it is so severely limited and he begins to cheat. Anybody who has crash dieted can remember a week or two of pleasing and satisfying weight loss followed by a leveling out period, beginning just when the deprivation of the diet begins to have its psychological effect. Very soon the dieter begins to eat more, and the adjusted body easily replaces the lost weight.

In some cases, with some of the more bizarre diets, the body will actually break down its lean tissue reserves before its fat reserves. Therefore, the weight loss that you first notice doesn't even represent loss of fat, but loss of lean protein and muscle. It is therefore apparent that all fad diet plans lack a certain amount of logic, and in the long run can be expected to fail.

Your Inherited Food Desires and
Their Effect on Heart Health

A look at human evolution will help illustrate what a balanced diet would be. The early ape men were gatherers of such foods as fruits and vegetables. They ate meat only occasionally, for they were not skilled hunters such as the predatory leopards and tigers. Predatory animals are adapted physiologically to digest an essentially meat diet, just as they are developed to hunt for it. The beginning of the story of intelligent man and advanced civilization is marked, not by an improvement in hunting skills, but by the development of agriculture! Man could now provide his food in a more reliable way, but it was still vegetables, especially grain, that formed the basic diet.

Grains are the source of vegetable oils—the same oils we have been talking about in this book. So you see, it is man's natural state to eat this type of diet. It is true that we always ate some meat, for our ancestors domesticated animals for dairy and slaughter purposes, but the staple food was always wheat, rice, corn, or some similar grain. Taken together, the grain, vegetables, meat, and dairy products provided a balanced diet that is the proper intake for a human animal. It is our responsibility to restore and preserve that balance so that we eat proper proportions of all foods. From this reasoning you can deduce that any imbalance is wrong—even those that may claim to be healthful.

The Only Reasonable Way to Lose Weight

The only reasonable way to lose weight is to eat proper proportions of fats, carbohydrates, and proteins, but in smaller amounts. If your total calorie intake drops below 2,000 calories a day, you will begin to lose weight. At 1,800 calories per day you will lose weight moderately, at 1,200 calories per day you will lose weight rather quickly, and 800 or 900 calories a day is what is referred to as a severe diet with rapid weight loss. It stands to reason that the more severe the diet, the most rapid the weight loss, but the harder it is to maintain the diet.

How to Keep the Excess Weight Off Your Body

Many people who have dieted are disappointed to see how easy it is to re-gain the lost weight. An explanation of why this happens can help you avoid this problem. Scientists have learned that during periods of excessive food intake, the body will make a new fat storage cell and fill it with fat, something like the way bees make a honeycomb cell and fill it with honey. At some time in the future if the person loses weight, the fat will be removed from the cell but the shell-like structure of the cell will remain for many months. If the dieter then abandons his diet and again consumes an excess amount of food, it is a relatively simple matter for the body to fill the storage cell with fat. If, on the other hand, he has maintained his lower weight for four to six months, that fat cell will be destroyed and absorbed. It is then more difficult for the body to make a new storage cell and fill it with fat. It therefore becomes more difficult to re-gain weight if you overeat only once in a while, for example, at a party or during a weekend out of town. Thus, a little extra perseverance with your diet will pay off and allow you to relax later on.

The Effect of Weight Reduction on Your Heart

Dieting to lose weight is a relatively short-term affair, but dieting to protect your heart is a lifetime commitment. If you are obese, you should lose weight and you should do so by counting calories. You can eat anything you want (in terms of calories) provided that at the end of the day your net total intake is below the number you have set. For example, if you choose a rich food for lunch, you must balance it by being more strict with your other meals on that day.

One Businessman's Problem

One particular patient, Mr. L., found it hard to cut down on his lunches because he was often meeting clients to combine business with lunch. It became increasingly difficult to keep his midday meal low enough in calories, so he and his family decided they would all use lunch as the main meal and supper became a more modest meal, enabling them all to maintain the proper balance. Other people might not be happy with that arrangement, but the lesson is the same for all. It involves the ability to plan. You can have a high-calorie food any time you want, but you must "pay" for it by combining it with a low-calorie food. The whole process can be compared to budgeting your paycheck. If you spend too much in one place, you will have much less to go around for other things, so the most satisfying plan is to spend intelligently everywhere with very few splurges. Dieting is the same—you have a certain daily resource of about 2,200 calories. If you "spend" too much in one place, you won't have enough to go around comfortably. Therefore, you must plan to distribute your "allowance" properly.

The best way to proceed is to obtain a small vest-pocket-sized calorie counter, and keep it with you all day. Everything you eat should be recorded with a running total of calories kept for each day. In this manner you can make sure that you don't accidentally go over your limit. Once you have brought your weight to the desired level, it should be easy to maintain it while following the unsaturated fat plan in this book. But remember, an unsaturated fat is just as rich as a saturated fat in terms of calories and therefore in terms of weight gain. The only difference between the two fats is in their effect on your arteries and heart. However, by decreasing your saturated fat intake, you will almost certainly decrease your total fat intake. Many people find weight reduction to be less of a problem while on a low-fat, low-cholesterol diet. They are able to maintain their proper weight with little extra effort, whereas previously they were not successful despite several repeated attempts at dieting.

Remember that an ordinary reducing diet will not give you the protection you want for your heart unless you not only lower your fat intake, but also substitute some unsaturated fat for saturated fat.

With this general background in mind, you should now ask, "Where do I start?" The answer begins with the next several chapters of instructions, and ends on the recipe pages, where you will find specific recipes designed for your family's health and happiness.

Chapter 8 • How to Shop for Low-Fat Foods

We have shown you evidence that proper eating can prevent heart attacks and that an improved diet can be possible while you continue to enjoy most of the food you like. This is possible because much of the "bad" in your food is hidden and can easily be replaced with healthier ingredients. This process of substitution is the essence of this book.

If you are to adapt successfully to this new way of eating, you must start with grocery shopping; in order to cook properly, you need the correct ingredients. For most people this means that you must acquire new habits in food buying. The idea is to avoid buying products containing the harmful fats, when you can just as easily buy safe ones. There is often quite a difference in the contents of foods that at first appear to be similar.

How to Read Labels on Packages

On shopping day, put on your glasses and read the fine print on each package. Ingredients are listed in decreasing order of quantity. For example, if there is more flour than sugar in a product, the word "flour" will appear before the word "sugar" on the label.

While it is best not to buy a product that contains any unhealthy fats, there are, of course, exceptions. Some foods contain very small amounts of fat, and their use may be quite acceptable. For example, the small amount of shortening in dry cookies or pretzels would not disqualify them from a low-fat diet. Since you can get a rough idea of the fat content of any product just by noting where the fat is listed with respect to the other ingredients, you can often make a decision on this basis. The most common ingredients to avoid are shortening, cheese, chocolate, and hydrogenated oils.

Hydrogenated Foods

Beware of the word *hydrogenated!* It means that the oil has been changed from unsaturated to saturated, and is therefore no longer healthy. *Hydrogenated fat* is often called hardened, partially hardened, or hydrogenated vegetable oil. These phrases mean that the oil that started out as a safe, healthy, unsaturated fat, is now a harmful one and should be avoided.

How to Spot Misleading Descriptions on Labels

Many other pitfalls exist because of the descriptive phrases used by food processors. For example, when vegetable oil is listed on a label, how do you decide if it is coconut oil or corn oil? The difference between the two is so great that they aren't even in the same league, and there is no way you can make an intelligent decision without some additional information. Beware of claims such as "special process oil" or "low fat." They tell you nothing. These words are often used to fool people who are not alert. A vague term, such as "low fat" could be camouflage for hydrogenated oils or even for shortening.

You need specific information and should get it by phoning or writing the manufacturer if necessary. You can often contact the food processor and ask to speak to the plant chemist or engineer. He will give you details on the fat content of the specific product. At first it may seem that you are constantly writing or phoning your local food suppliers. Actually, a few such inquiries when you start should take care of almost all your questions.

Many undesirable fats exist where you would not expect to find them. For example, frozen fried fish sticks are often fried in lard. Just compare the amount of saturated fat in these with the same fish fried in oil. The value of eating the fish is lost if the frying is done in lard. The taste may be the same, but the effect on your heart is not.

Often commercial substitutions are made for reasons of economy or with manufacturing process in mind, and show little concern for health or heart disease. Once you have learned to read the labels with sophistication, you will be able to avoid things that say "vegetable fat" because that is not enough information. A little knowledge will enable you to make the proper choice in shopping and food preparation; sometimes switching brands is all that is necessary.

Edible Oils

As we discussed in chapter 4, fats can be divided into two main types, saturated and unsaturated. The unsaturated fats, such as vegetable oils, are the beneficial ones and are usually in liquid form. The saturated fats found in butter, meat, and shortening are usually solid at room temperature; these are the unhealthy fats. Exceptions to this liquid-solid rule do exist. For example, coconut oil, although a liquid, has an exceptionally high saturated fat content. Because of its long shelf life, coconut oil is often used in commercially prepared foods such as whipped toppings, convenience foods, and imitation dairy products. Read the label carefully to alert yourself. Unfortunately, however, very often the type of oil may not be specified.

The oil you use in cooking and baking can be left to personal preference providing it is one of the following—corn, soybean, cotton-seed, or safflower. While olive oil and peanut oil are not saturated and therefore not harmful, neither are they highly unsaturated—thus they do not lower blood cholesterol. They should not be used to supply the needed unsaturated fats in our diet. If olive oil is a favorite in your household, use it, for example, in salads, but use the other oils in all cooking and baking to maintain the needed unsaturated fat balance.

Hydrogenated Margarine

Margarine is vegetable oil that has been hardened to a saturated form to resemble butter. This is accomplished by the hydrogenation process described earlier. Liquid corn oil, when made into solid mar-garine, has nothing added to it—it is only the chemical process of hydrogenation that turns the liquid into solid, saturated fat.

Margarine occupies the central position on a scale that has butter and saturated fat at one end, and oil and unsaturated fat at the other. Margarine can be highly saturated or partly unsaturated. With the growth of interest in low-fat diets, many new low-fat margarines are appearing.

The newer, whipped types of margarine rank fairly close to oils in their unsaturated content. Even these, however, are not as unsatu-rated as oil and should be considered only as halfway products in terms of health.

Margarine served in most restaurants belongs at the saturated end of the scale and is really nothing more than synthetic butter with all the disadvantages of butter. Other types of special margarines, such as low-salt margarine, do exist. These may be specially modified, but since it is not the saturated fat content that is changed, we need not consider them for our purpose.

Some low-calorie margarines are whipped with air and water, which reduces the fat content but does not change the type of fat. It is the amount of unsaturated fat compared to the amount of saturated fat in each margarine that is really essential. The best examples of the low-saturated-fat margarines are often called "special" margarines. These contain about 45 percent unsaturated fat and 15 to 20 percent saturated fat. (The remaining part is monounsaturated, which can be considered neutral.) Chiffon, Fleishmann's, and Mazola are some common brands that fall into the preceding category.

How to Compare Margarine Brands

Other local or new brands may be available in your area. The best way to compare different brands is to divide the saturated fat content into the unsaturated fat content. For example, if Brand X contains 50 percent unsaturated fat and 20 percent saturated fat, the result is 50/20 or 2.5. The higher this number, the better the margarine.

If you cannot find out the percentages, you should select brands that list liquid oil as the first ingredient. Remember, most "special" margarines are sold in tubs, but not all tub margarines are "special."

Beware of false advertising. There are many appealing, but untrue, advertising claims that read "more polyunsaturates penny for penny and pound for pound." Such statements are nonsense. What do they mean? Madison Avenue likes to jump on a bandwagon, even if the truth is not served.

Dairy Products

Milk—Skim and Whole

Skim milk and whole milk both contain exactly the same amount of protein, minerals, and vitamins. The only difference is that in skim milk the fat has been removed. Since milk is such a staple food in our normal diet, changing to skim milk is a big step toward cutting down on fat intake. If your family complains about drinking skim milk, change over gradually. Try mixing whole and skim milk together, and gradually decrease the whole milk and increase the skim milk until you are using only skim. We have never known anyone who could not switch over, and we have never known anyone who could switch back once they became accustomed to skim milk.

Skim milk is less than one-tenth of one percent fat (99.9 percent fat free) or it is not skim milk. Other types of low-fat milk that are not as safe may be called "modified milk," "fortified milk," "less than 1% fat," or "99% fat free." There are enough types in the average supermarket to confuse even the most wary shopper. When you see the words, "low fat," look closer and see if it really is less than one-tenth of one percent. Some low-fat milk is 2 percent fat and that is twenty times more fat than true skim milk. For economical reasons, we often use powdered skim milk, especially for cooking and baking.

We have found that the better-quality powders are worth the extra money because they usually have a more natural flavor.

Yogurt

Yogurt is a marvelous dairy product that you can use frequently and it is now commercially available as 99 percent fat free. Check the brands in your neighborhood and try to buy the low-fat ones, although even regular yogurt is relatively low in fat.

Cheese

Cottage cheese is the main type of cheese to use because of its low fat content. If your family really prefers hard cheese, there are skim milk types on the market. This means that part of the milk used in their processing is skim milk, but the rest of the milk is either whole milk or cream. Since some skim milk is used, these cheeses will have less saturated fat than regular cheese and should be used in place of them. Some contain about 7 percent fat, compared to 30 to 70 percent for regular cheese, so the difference is significant. But do check on each brand since the fat content will vary.

Cottage cheese should form the basic or staple portion of your cheese consumption. If you are using large amounts of cottage cheese for cooking or baking, it is better to buy the skim-milk or fat-free type. This cheese comes in various styles of curd size and liquid content. If the cheese is too dry, add a little skim milk, or if it is too wet, drain and then sieve or blend until smooth. Consistencies vary from type to type, so use your judgment to achieve the final result you prefer.

On rare occasions you may want to flavor some food such as macaroni with a real "cheesy" taste that is not available in skim milk variety. For this purpose, buy the strongest Cheddar, grate it, and then use very little so that you can have maximum flavor with minimum fat content.

Artificial Fat Can Cause Real Heart Disease

Imitation dairy products, such as artificial cream for coffee (both frozen and powdered), artificial sour cream, artificial cheese, artificial ice cream, thick shakes, and frozen puddings are often labeled very clearly "no butterfat, no cholesterol." But what these products often do contain is coconut oil—a much more saturated fat than even butter! We consider this to be deceptive and the federal government is now working on this problem with an improved "Truth in Labeling Law."

Toppings

Whipped toppings, whether in packages, in aerosol cans, or in frozen form should not be used because of their high saturated fat content. See our recipe in chapter 19 so that you can prepare your own at an incredibly lower cost and with no loss of flavor.

How to Buy Meat

Be careful to buy only lean cuts of fresh or frozen unprepared meat. Do not buy canned or frozen cooked meats since there is no way of knowing how much or what type of fat they contain. Also avoid hot dogs, sausages, salami, bolognas, and pressed luncheon meats. The law allows for a high fat content in hot dogs and the manufacturer usually takes full advantage of this allowance. Search for modified brands of frankfurters, salami, and sausages. These are becoming available in decreased saturated fat and cholesterol versions, but most communities do not have this type of food product as yet. Organ meats are high in cholesterol and should be eaten sparingly. See the chapter on meat for more specific hints on shopping and preparation.

How to Buy Fish

Fish is an excellent source both of protein and unsaturated fat. It should be used frequently in place of the meat that plays such a large part in the American diet. The variety of fish available to us today is almost endless. We can buy fresh, frozen, smoked, or canned fish. Shellfish occupy an ambiguous position since they are high in cholesterol but also high in unsaturated fat, so eat them, but sparingly.

It is a good idea to keep cans of fish on your pantry shelf for a quick meal. Check the oil that the fish is packed in because the ones canned in olive oil are not as beneficial as the others packed in other vegetable oils.

Frozen fish that has been coated or prepared in a batter should be checked very carefully; most manufacturers use shortening or hydrogenated oils in the preparation. Look through the section on fish for a variety of recipes and hints on how to prepare your own.

How to Buy Poultry

Chicken and turkey (except the prebasted type that has been injected with coconut oil) are excellent for our purposes. They are readily available, versatile, and usually economical. We discuss many ways to prepare these in the poultry section. While the light meat is leaner than the dark meat, trimmed dark meat is still very lean. Cornish hens and squabs are acceptable and offer a nice change. Do not buy either duck or goose; these are simply too fatty and no method of preparation or trimming can alter this.

Chicken and turkey can go a long way in helping to economize on food purchases and in minimizing your work. For example, there are many paella rice mixes on the market that contain no fat in themselves. With the addition of chicken, fish, and vegetables, they make a hearty dish. The mix sits on the shelf until you have leftovers, then just take it out, add the leftovers, and you have a quick, easy, and economical meal.

Eggs

While saturated fat and cholesterol are present in the yolk of an egg, they are completely absent from the white, which is almost pure protein. Therefore, we try to use more egg white and less yolk in all our cooking and baking. You may want to purchase powdered egg white. It is available in some retail stores.

These powdered whites are somewhat inconvenient to use since they must be prepared in advance. Our experience has been that it is easier and not any more expensive to use the desired amount of whites and simply throw out the yolks. It may seem wasteful at first, but you will not mind if you remember that it is better for you if the yolk clogs the drain instead of your arteries.

Now there is available a new product containing egg whites, but no egg yolk. The yolk is replaced by a no-cholesterol vegetable substitute that is safe to eat. Although you cannot make soft-boiled eggs from this frozen product, you can use it for scrambled eggs, omelets, and in cooking and baking. The brand name is Egg Beaters, made by Fleishmann's.

Various Packaged Food Products

We were quite surprised to learn that one of the leading brands of *pudding mix* contains coconut oil (highly saturated), while a second leading brand that tastes just as good does not.

Commercial crackers, with the exception of plain soda crackers, are usually quite high in fat. Therefore, we recommend the use of bread sticks, melba toast, matzo, party rye, or party pumpernickle.

The party breads, found in the dairy case, are very thin and make excellent dippers or cracker replacements. They can also be dried slowly in the oven to make melba toast.

Dehydrated products such as *potato mixes,* to which you can add oil yourself, are usually safe and acceptable. Again, read the labels carefully.

More and more *cakes and muffin mixes* are appearing on the market. As of now, very few are made with unsaturated fat. Angel food cake is the only one we have found to be safe. We can only suggest that you keep checking the ingredients in each new type that appears; perhaps in time there will be more acceptable mixes available. A letter to some of the larger manufacturers might help speed this up.

Note: Do not become dependent on mixes and prepared products. We have found that the extra time it takes to prepare your own tempting sauce for a vegetable or pasta dish is only minutes. Although the prepackaged noodle or rice preparations look inviting, they are only slightly faster to prepare, often contain a great deal of forbidden fat, and are very much more expensive. Get into the habit of preparing your own.

Cocoa and Chocolate

The difference between cocoa and chocolate is that cocoa is the residue left when cocoa butter is removed from the chocolate. The cocoa that is left is relatively free of saturated fat and can be used in moderate amounts. In some supermarkets low-fat cocoa is available, which is even better.

Chocolate-covered cookies are sometimes made with chocolate and sometimes made with cocoa. If they are a favorite with your family, buy the ones made with cocoa and use these only as an occasional treat.

Topping Off the Grocery List

—Always buy salad dressing types of mayonnaise rather than pure mayonnaise. The difference is that salad dressing contains less egg yolk than mayonnaise.
—Check the commercial liquid types of salad dressings to learn which type of oil they contain.
—The icing used in most commercial cookies is usually 50 percent shortening and should never be eaten.
—When choosing a brand of peanut butter, do not buy one that is *hydrogenated;* this means that the oils used have been hardened.

If the label says *homogenized,* this is fine since it only means that the oil does not separate. You can make your own peanut butter by blending shelled peanuts until they become smooth. A little peanut oil will make the peanut butter less sticky—use about two teaspoons per half cup of peanuts.

—There are soybean products containing little or no saturated fat that taste like crisp, crumbled bacon or pepperoni. These can be found under several brand names, such as Bac*Os or Pepr*Os. We use them frequently in sandwiches and pizzas.

—When buying salted nuts, buy only the dry-roasted type with no fat added. All plain, raw, shelled nuts are permissible.

—Imitation butter flavoring is available at your supermarket. Use it whenever you desire a buttery taste.

—Frozen T.V. dinners, precooked food, and vegetables frozen with butter and sauce must all be avoided since you cannot determine how much or what type of fat they contain.

How to Become a Sharp Food Buyer for Your Heart's Sake

Become smarter than the food manufacturers! Many commercial processes and substitutions work against the concepts embodied in this book. A flagrant example of how unwanted fat is forced on you is found in powdered orange drink and other fruit drinks that are becoming very popular. Some of these, for example, are heavily advertised as the drink the astronauts used on their space flights. How many people would even dream that the label on this (and other) fruit drinks reveals the presence of hydrogenated vegetable oil? Even though this amount is small, it ought to make every thinking person angry to be victimized this way. It should at least caution us to read labels when shopping.

Do not be discouraged by what may at first seem to be a lot of bother. There are certainly enough acceptable products available, but we must learn to recognize them. *Read the smallest print on each label.* At first this may be time consuming, but in no time at all you will learn to buy the healthiest food for your family and the end result will be well worth the effort.

SHOPPING GUIDE

All items appearing in "prepare at home" column should not be used if commercially prepared.

	Local Store	Prepare at Home	Do Not Use
Anchovies	X		
Avocado	X		
†Bacon: Canadian	X		
Bacon: regular			X
Bagel	X		
Barley	X		
Beans: baked vegetarian only	X		
†Beef: roasts, steaks, ground, stew, lean	X		
*Beef stroganoff		X	
Beer	X		
Beverages: alcoholic, carbonated, cider, tea, coffee, fruit flavored	X		
*Biscuits: mix and dough		X	
Bologna			X
Boston Brown Bread	X		
Bouillon and bouillon cubes	X		
Brains			X
*Bread: cake-type		X	
Bread crumbs and stuffing (plain)	X		
Bread: loaf, all kinds except rich breads and those containing egg yolks	X		
Bread: rich and egg-type			X
Bread sticks	X		
*Brownies		X	
Buttermilk (low fat)	X		
Butterscotch syrup		X	
Cake: angel food (unfrosted)	X		
Cake mixes: white, yellow, chocolate, spice			X
*Cakes: white, yellow, chocolate, spice, etc.		X	
*Candies: chocolate or fat-containing		X	
Candies: nonfat, hard (fruit drops, lollipops, etc.), jellies, mints, gum drops, licorice, glazed fruits, and nuts	X		
Catsup, chili sauce	X		
Caviar	X		
Cereals: all kinds	X		

* Recipe included
† Check grocery shopping

	Local Store	Prepare at Home	Do Not Use
*Cheese cake		X	
†Cheeses: cottage	X		
processed loaf			X
spreads		X	
Chicken: broilers and fryers	X		
*Chocolate candy		X	
Chocolate milk		X	
*Chocolate syrup		X	
*Chowder, clam: Boston-type or New England		X	
Chowder, clam: canned Manhattan	X		
Clams: canned, frozen, or fresh	X		
Cocktails (except those made with cream or egg)	X		
Cocoa	X		
Coconut			X
Coffee	X		
*Coffeecake		X	
*Commercially prepared foods; canned or frozen: braised beef and vegetables, chicken cacciatore, chopped chicken livers, roast beef slices, tuna Newburg, lasagna, etc.		X	
Concentrate for milk, skim	X		
Cookies (low-fat): animal crackers, arrowroot, vanilla wafers, ginger snaps, lemon snaps, fig bars	X		
*Cookies: rich		X	
*Corn bread and muffins		X	
Cornish game hens	X		
Cornmeal	X		
Cornstarch	X		
Crabmeat: canned, frozen, or fresh	X		
Cracker meal	X		
Crackers: graham, oyster, rye wafers, saltine, soda, melba toast, rusk	X		
Crackers: snack-type			X
Cream, coffee: powdered			X
skim milk powder	X		
Croutons		X	
*Cupcakes		X	
Dairy products: artificial			X
*Danish-type pastry—coffeecakes		X	
Dates	X		
*Dips		X	

* Recipe included
† Check grocery shopping

	Local Store	Prepare at Home	Do Not Use
Doughnuts: cake-type, frozen		X	
Duck			X
Dumplings		X	
*Eclairs		X	
Egg mix			X
Eggs: whole	X		
†Fats: cooking (see oil)	X		
Fish: canned, fresh, frozen, smoked	X		
Flavoring extracts	X		
Flour: all kinds	X		
Frankfurters (hot dogs)			X
*French toast		X	
Fried potatoes		X	
Frog legs (raw)	X		
*Frostings		X	
*Frozen deserts: vanilla, strawberry, chocolate, etc.		X	
Fruit: fruit juices, dried fruits	X		
Fruit toppings	X		
Game: venison, elk, etc.	X		
Game birds: quail, pheasant, etc.	X		
*Garlic bread		X	
Gefilte fish	X		
Gelatin: powder and dessert	X		
Gin	X		
Goose			X
Gravy		X	
†Ham (lean)	X		
Ham hocks			X
†Hamburger (lean)	X		
Heart: all kinds			X
Herbs: all kinds	X		
Honey	X		
*Ice cream (see frozen desserts)		X	
Jams, jellies, marmalades	X		
Kidneys			X

---

* Recipe included
† Check grocery shopping

	Local Store	Prepare at Home	Do Not Use
Lamb: roast, grillettes, cubed steak	X		
Liquor	X		
Liver	X		
Liver sausage			X
Lobster, lobster tail	X		
Luncheon meats: bologna, liver sausage, pressed meats			X
†Margarine	X		
Marshmallows, marshmallow whip	X		
Matzo (except those made with eggs)	X		
Mayonnaise (salad dressing type)	X		
*Meringue: shells or mix	X		
Milk: chocolate		X	
*Milk: shakes		X	
Milk: skim (liquid or powdered)	X		
Molasses	X		
*Muffins		X	
Mushroom soup		X	
Mustard	X		
Noodles	X		
Nuts: all kinds (dry-roasted or in shells)	X		
Oil: cooking or salad	X		
Olives	X		
Oysters: fresh, frozen, or canned	X		
*Paella		X	
Pancake mix	X		
Pastas: all kinds—lasagna, macaroni, noodles, spaghetti	X		
Pastas: cooked with sauce		X	
Pastries		X	
Peanut butter (nonhydrogenated)	X		
Pickles and relishes	X		
*Pies		X	
Pie fillings (fruit only)	X		
*Pie shells		X	
Pigs feet and tails			X
*Pizza		X	
Popcorn (ready to pop; avoid prepared type with fat added)	X		

* Recipe included
† Check grocery shopping

	Local Store	Prepare at Home	Do Not Use
†Pork, cured: (see ham, sausage, Canadian bacon)	X		
Pork, fresh: roasts, steaks, cutlets, grillettes	X		
Pork sausage (links)			X
Potatoes: all except fried or those with cheese added	X		
Potato chips			X
Potatoes: French-fried		X	
*Poultry: chicken, turkey, Cornish game hen	X		
duck, goose			X
Pretzels	X		
†Pudding powders (except chocolate and coconut)	X		
Rabbit	X		
Rennet powder	X		
Rice: all kinds	X		
†Roasts: beef, lamb, pork, veal	X		
Rolls: hamburger, hard, wiener, soft (not sweet or rich butter-type)	X		
*Rolls: sweet, coffeecake		X	
*Salad dressing: dry mixes (except cheese-type)	X		
Salad dressing: French, Italian	X		
*Salad dressing: mayonnaise-type	X	X	
Salmon	X		
Salt and seasoned salts	X		
Salt pork			X
Sardines	X		
Sauces (seasoning for gravies, steak sauce, soy, Worcestershire, catsup, chili, horseradish)	X		
*Sauces: meat		X	
*Sauces, prepared mixes: lemon, sour cream, white, spaghetti		X	
Sausage, pork			X
*Shellfish: canned, fresh, or frozen	X		
Sherbet and ices (low-fat)	X		
Short ribs			X
*Shrimp: canned, fresh, or frozen	X		
Skim milk (liquid or powder)	X		
*Soup, cream of mushroom		X	

* Recipe included
† Check grocery shopping

	Local Store	Prepare at Home	Do Not Use
*Soups, creamed		X	
Soups, low-fat: beef noodle, chicken noodle or chicken rice, chicken gumbo, tomato, tomato rice, vegetable, vegetable-beef	X		
*Sour cream		X	
Spaghetti	X		
Spaghetti sauce, canned: meatless	X		
*Spaghetti sauce: meat		X	
Spareribs			X
Spices: all types	X		
*Spreads and dips (see cheese spreads)		X	
Steaks, beef: cube, strip loin, tenderloin, top round, top sirloin	X		
*Steaks, ham: fresh and smoked	X		
Stewing hens			X
Sugar: all types	X		
Sweetbreads			X
*Sweet rolls		X	
Syrup (no butter added)	X		
*Syrup: butterscotch and chocolate		X	
Tapioca	X		
Tomato: aspic, sauce	X		
Tongue			X
Tuna fish	X		
*Turkey (not deep basted or prebasted)	X		
*T.V. dinners		X	
Veal: roast, cutlets, chops, grillettes	X		
*Vegetables and vegetable juice: all fresh, frozen, or canned without added fat, meat, cheese or sauces	X		
Vinegar	X		
Waffles		X	
Wheat germ	X		
*Whipped topping		X	
Whiskey	X		
Wine	X		
Yeast	X		
Yogurt (made with skim milk)	X		

* Recipe included
† Check grocery shopping

Chapter 9 · Easy Menu Planning for the Heart's Sake

Once convinced of the health benefits of low-fat foods, the housewife must now take over the planning. It is her duty to introduce her husband and her children to a *new way of eating!* This can easily be done using the extensive recipe section of this book, but a short discussion on how to use the recipes may prove helpful.

The meals must be planned with our previously discussed concepts in mind: you will be using our recipes and revising your own to cut down saturated fat and cholesterol to healthier levels. This is not a difficult or complicated task. You don't have to count how much fat is involved—there are no calculations—just follow our suggestions to be sure that you are saving your family from the many serious effects of too much fat.

To help you select recipes and plan meals, the following general principles should be followed.

Meat, Poultry, and Fish

A source of protein should be served at each meal. While protein can be found in meat, fish, or poultry, a greater reliance on fish and poultry instead of meat will provide more protein with less fat. Red meat such as steak and beef should not be served more than three times per week because of its high fat content. Dried peas, beans, nuts, and peanut butter are high in protein and can also count toward a serving in this category.

Cheese

Cheese made from skim milk is another good source of protein. Some fat is present in these cheeses, but all in all, they can be used in our plan. Many families rely on cheese-based meals as an economical and quick-to-prepare method of obtaining protein.

Low-fat cheese is available in several common types: cottage cheese, mozzarella cheese, and yellow brick cheese. Regular cheese has an even higher fat content than most beef. Therefore, if used, it must be counted as a substitute for your beef allowance.

Skim milk cheeses give you nearly as much protein and much less fat than beef. Make good use of this high-protein food in anything from a grilled cheese sandwich to an 'au gratin" dish of your choice.

Skim Milk

Skim milk is almost a wonder food and should be consumed daily —two cups a day for adults and four cups a day for children. It may be used in a pudding, in sauces, and of course as a beverage. Buttermilk made from skim milk is a refreshing drink and is especially tasty when poured over berries or when used in the preparation of pancakes and some baked goods.

Remember that milk is a prime source of protein. It should be clearly understood that skim milk has no less protein or minerals than whole milk—the only difference is that the fat has been removed. We remember a neighbor who forced her child to finish a huge glass of whole milk at every meal—for nourishment! This is an excellent example of the lack of understanding and common sense that exists in this country. The child was overweight to start with, and did not need the extra calories contained in the whole milk. A more important consideration, however, was the effect of all the extra fat he had consumed. There was really no justification for this mother to force or even allow this much unnecessary fat in her child's diet.

We know now that the seeds of later heart disease are sown in early childhood. It is far better to use the healthier product—skim milk—especially when you realize you are giving up fat and calories, not protein.

Yogurt

Flavored yogurt is a delicious snack or dessert and unflavored yogurt makes an acceptable substitute for sour cream, which is taboo. However, don't forget our recipe for "sour cream" made from cottage cheese. (See page 88.) Use either this or yogurt whenever you would normally use regular sour cream—for example, with berries, bananas, vegetables, in cooking, or as a base for some delicious dips.

Eggs

Do not use eggs as a main course since your recommended allowance for egg yolks is limited to four a week. Since whole eggs are often used in the preparation of desserts, breads, crackers, and noodles, you will quickly reach your limit by a normal consumption of these products. If two egg yolks are used in a cake and there are eight portions, one person will consume one-quarter of a yolk. In some recipes we eliminate even half a yolk. This does not seem like much of a saving, but why use even a small amount of saturated fat if it is not necessary? Every little bit counts!

Remember, all the saturated fat in eggs is in the yolk and none at all is in the white, which is a good source of protein. Use as many whites as you wish. Many of our recipes for mousses, icings, and gelatin desserts are prepared with only the whites.

Vegetables and Fruit

Four or more servings of vegetables, fruit, and pure fruit juices should be in every daily plan. It is a good idea to include citrus or another fruit or vegetable high in vitamin C. In addition, one vegetable should be of the dark green or yellow variety, such as pumpkin, sweet potato, carrot, spinach, broccoli, or cabbage. These supply vitamin A. Although fat content is not a problem in vegetables, we mention them just to make sure a balanced food intake is achieved.

Whole Grains and Enriched Breads and Cereals

You should have three servings a day of enriched breads or cereals. See our recipe sections for some delicious and healthy muffins and breads.

Doing It the Easy Way

Menu planning need not be a complex procedure. Every housewife does some kind of menu planning, even though she may not call it that. After all, she has to decide what to serve at each meal. It is not our intent to make you into a dietitian with slide rule, measuring cup, and kitchen scale. The guidelines you have just read merely emphasize certain aspects that can be implemented with a little extra thought.

Every family consumes some meat, some vegetables, and some dairy products. Basically, you should plan meals to include less beef and more of the other protein sources as described. If you served a beef meal yesterday, choose a recipe from the poultry or fish section for today. Try the recipes in this book to make use of the ways we have found to avoid undesirable fats. Many of the recipes even have the vegetables included. Try the salmon with zucchini or the baked veal and eggplant for a healthy main course.

You would not survive long on a diet devoid of fats, so you

should not feel guilty every time you serve a meal containing some source of fat. Try to eliminate most hard or saturated fat, which is found in coconut oil, butter, whole milk, cream, cheese, most artificial dairy products, red meat, and chocolate. However, you cannot avoid saturated fat completely. *Our primary objective is to increase your unsaturated or soft fat intake and to decrease your saturated or hard fat intake.*

Practically speaking, oil should be consumed daily, either in the form of salad dressings or in cooking and baking. The easiest and most pleasant way of doing this is to continue cooking most of the food your family is accustomed to eating; just change the type of fat. Using our recipes or methods of substitution for food you generally eat will accomplish this for you. You will actually change your fat intake unconsciously—the recipes are planned that way. For example, our version of beef stroganoff or of creamed soup is a world apart from your old recipe in fat content, but the taste is the same.

Breakfast

The typical American breakfast is usually one of two types—both bad. The first is the bacon and egg breakfast, and the other is sweet roll or donuts and coffee—both are loaded with fat and have little nutrition.

Each day should begin with a hearty breakfast that includes fruit, bread or cereal, and skim milk. These basics can be served in many forms.

The fruits may include fresh fruit, stewed fruit, or fruit juice. The breads or cereals may be substituted by pancakes, waffles, muffins, and even French toast (if it is prepared from our recipe). The skim milk may be used as a beverage, on cereals, or in coffee. If you want to make "cream" for your hot cereal or coffee, you can do so by adding three tablespoons of skim milk powder to eight ounces of skim milk and refrigerate for a few hours before using.

For those who like a larger breakfast, you can include fish, such as herring, kippers, or smoked salmon. In other words, you can eat a large, nourishing meal and still avoid the old repetitious fatty, buttery breakfast.

If you like coffeecakes, you may be disappointed to learn that they are full of butter. Don't despair! This book includes many recipes for such treats as johnny cake, coffeecake, muffins, and cinnamon rolls, all prepared with no butter and a minimal number of eggs. These make delicious breakfast changes and are much healthier than the traditional bacon and eggs fare.

A skimpy or inadequate breakfast is a bad habit from at least two points of view. In the first place, it leaves you hungry by midmorning and sets you up for an overindulgent coffee break. The available snack is usually donuts, cake, potato chips, or a chocolate bar—all unnecessary and unhealthy. You will then eat more than you should and you will find you gain weight easier. A big mistake that dieters often make is to try to "save" calories (or fat) at breakfast, and end up by losing ground at midmorning or lunch time.

There is even another reason to avoid this pitfall. Your body is not designed to function well on an all-or-nothing energy supply. It is unhealthy to go to work with an empty stomach, have a midmorning snack, then lunch, and a heavy dinner. It is much better, from the point of the body's ability to metabolize its food, to consume your daily calories in evenly spaced amounts, rather than at one or two huge meals.

Lunch

Lunch can be simpler than dinner, but hearty, too. You might start with soup or juice, accompanied by varieties of salads or sandwiches. This is an excellent time to serve fish or whip up a casserole of last night's leftovers. Our chapter on appetizers and lunch dishes should give you many new ideas. You may conclude the meal with a dessert and a beverage.

Businessman's Lunch

Many people now carry an attaché case to work with a polyunsaturated lunch! One husband we know solved the problem of a wife who was not anxious to take on the added work of packing a lunch each day; he paid her the cost of his lunch. Now she protects her husband's heart and has additional spending money to show for her effort.

If you prefer to have lunch at a restaurant, you can still eat well within safe and reasonable limits. See chapter 11 for specific advice on eating out.

Dinner

Dinner is usually the main meal of the day and is looked forward to by the family, so plan carefully. You can avoid the repetition of fish or chicken dishes by using our international variety of recipes.

Be sure to balance your fats at each meal. For example, when serving a red meat, serve only an eggless or fruit dessert. When serving a fish or poultry meal, you can serve a dessert that contains some egg yolk. Try serving soup first or an extra vegetable so that your meat portions may be smaller and your family will not feel hungry. Make liberal use of the many pickles and relishes available to add variety.

Convenience Foods

Frozen, precooked meals including T.V. dinners should be carefully checked for hidden hard fats. Commercially prepared foods, such as stuffed peppers, cheese manicotti, lasagna, baked stuffed potatoes, fish sticks, and so on, are all filled with saturated fat and are expensive as well. Simple recipes are included in this book that will enable you to make and freeze your own, thereby saving not only your arteries, but also your grocery money. The point is that these dishes can be enjoyed without eating dangerous fat—all you have to do is learn how to prepare them yourself and not rely on commercial varieties.

Remember, all types of fats are present in all food, but the proportions vary. After using this book, and living with our method for a while, you will easily learn to classify a food by its fat content— saturated or unsaturated. This will enable you to plan meals that contain a higher proportion of unsaturated fats.

You Can Teach Old Recipes New Tricks

The recipes in this book are the ones our friends and families like the most. Many are old favorites that began as butter- or fat-based offenders, but have since been reformed into healthy food.

You can learn to substitute soft fats for hard fats, trim your meats carefully, and throw away extra egg yolk. Many helpful hints on how to adapt your own recipes are discussed in the various sections, so don't hesitate to add to your collection with your own family's favorites.

Chapter 10 · Proper Use of
Your Freezer or Refrigerator
Freezing Compartment

One of the major results of your new approach to eating is that you will be serving much less commercially packaged food and more thoughtfully prepared home-cooked dishes. Because you prepare the food yourself, you have full control over what you feed your family, and can therefore reduce their fat intake. You also have the added dividend of reducing your food costs. Compare your cost of preparing chicken with that of a T.V. dinner. More important, commercial, pre-cooked meals contain cheaper cuts of meat with high fat content, and gravies and sauces made from shortening or fat drippings.

Proper use of your freezer can significantly reduce the time involved in food preparation. When you are cooking or baking, it is wise to make more than you need, regardless of the size of your family, and then freeze in one-meal servings. You will be surprised at the savings in both time and money when you prepare your own food; you will also be delighted when you can serve your family healthy homemade "T.V. dinners" on busy days.

The freezer can be used for many purposes—to cook ahead so as to save time for busy days, to utilize leftovers for future meals, or to prepare food when the price is right.

Ease in Freezing

Rather than freeze in plastic containers, which take up so much room, we find plastic wrap or small plastic bags much more convenient for wrapping food. Plastic does not tear as foil sometimes does, it is transparent and thus does not need labeling, and the food keeps well.

One useful trick when freezing hamburger, chicken or veal patties, or raw chicken pieces is to freeze flat on a cookie sheet, un-wrapped, then place in a plastic bag for storage. This method of quick freezing will prevent pieces of food from sticking to each other in the bag. They can then be removed individually for use when needed.

Soups

Soups freeze very well. It takes only a little additional effort to prepare an extra amount, so use your largest pot and freeze some for cold, rainy days. If you have toddlers, freeze homemade soup in single servings for lunch.

Vegetables

Make good use of the freezer for vegetable dishes. You may cook the vegetables for our vegetable fried rice, for example, in large amounts and then freeze one-meal portions. That way you won't have to cook the vegetables each time, losing both vitamins and flavor. Just defrost and toss them into the rice. Many vegetable dishes freeze well, for example, ratatouille, potato pancakes, carrot pudding, and fritters (all described in the recipe section). These can be called upon to fill out your menu on short notice if you have them ready in your freezer.

Desserts

All the cookies, squares, and most of our cakes are excellent candidates for the freezer. It is a good idea to keep a variety of frozen baked goodies on hand so that you won't be tempted to buy the forbidden ones when you haven't time to bake. Remember, when freezing cakes, that an uniced cake will keep longer than an iced one.

All the breads, such as the banana-nut bread or date loaf, can be sliced when cool and frozen in plastic bags. Remove only as many slices as needed. They will thaw at room temperature in a few minutes —faster than you can perk the coffee—so there will be no reason to buy the more expensive and unhealthy frozen cakes.

If you are serving pudding or a plain piece of cake, you can garnish it with our frozen whipped topping. This topping can be kept frozen and is ready for instant use.

How to Save Your Heart and Your Money

As you can see, efficient use of your freezer has two advantages. First, and most important, it is healthier to prepare your own food. Second, it is cheaper to prepare your own food, and in these days of rising costs, who isn't anxious to save money?

In the recipe sections you will see that nearly all your favorite foods can be made with little or no saturated fat, unlike the same food commercially prepared, which is loaded with fat. It is up to you to refuse to accept this imposition by the food industry. Eat food made the way it should and can be made, and enjoy the satisfaction of preparing your own to safeguard the health of your family.

Chapter 11 • How to Order
When Eating Out

This section on eating out is included to help you maintain your new goals when away from home. I remember the case of Mr. T. whose wife worked diligently and faithfully with our plan. However, his blood cholesterol level did not decrease. After discussing the situation, it became apparent that he was following the diet plan at home for dinner, but neglecting it at all other times. It turned out that he left home early in the morning without breakfast. He then ate a Danish pastry type of breakfast downtown and an unhealthy lunch at a restaurant near his office. He needed guidance to prevent him from undoing all the good his wife accomplished at home. We told him how to order a healthy breakfast at a restaurant. With a little more instruction on how to order lunch when eating out, he soon became an enthusiastic example of success with the cholesterol-lowering program.

Eating out properly is not really difficult, but you will have to understand a few basic concepts about the difference between restaurant food and healthier homemade food.

If you use this book successfully, your family will be eating a wide variety of foods that would seem to be out of place on a low-fat diet, such as chicken à la king, beef stroganoff, and chocolate cake. They may not realize that it is the preparation that makes these safe to eat, and that the same food ordered in a restaurant would be harmful.

In other words, the housewife must remember to inform her family that many foods found in restaurants are not prepared with the same methods and consideration as at home. For example, when you see chicken à la king on a menu, you must realize that it is made with cream or whole milk, and that a commercial chocolate cake is usually made with chocolate and butter or shortening. You must learn to recognize which are acceptable foods and which are not.

Sometimes you can have your restaurant meals modified by a simple request. For example, have fish prepared without butter, or vegetables served without the sauce. You will find that most restaurants are more than willing to accommodate. Remember though, that some things cannot be modified. There is no way to obtain a "safe" chocolate cake in a restaurant—save that for home. Because of the many choices on most menus, you can order well for all courses and stay within our scheme. To give you a framework on which to base your choices when eating out, the following paragraphs offer hints and guidelines.

Breads

Rye, white, whole wheat, and French commercial loaves are all acceptable, as are English muffins, melba toast, and rye crisps. The main thing to avoid is buttery rolls. At breakfast be sure to order your toast dry (no additional butter) and spread it yourself with cottage cheese, jam, or jelly. For other meals, a good restaurant will serve rolls that are usually fresh and warm enough to be enjoyed without butter. Anything less than that isn't worth filling up on, with butter or without.

Cereals

You can order either dry or hot cereals. When adding milk to cereals, two percent fat milk is usually available if skim milk is not, and should be used instead of whole milk. If you can't obtain either skim or two percent fat milk, use a very small amount of whole milk. Never use "half and half" since one of these halves is cream; this combination is even higher in saturated fat than whole milk.

Soups

Soups should be either jellied consommé or clear, hot broth. Most clear soups have had the fat removed. Thick soups should be avoided in restaurants even if they appear to have no fat on the surface. You may not be able to see the fat, but it is often there. Creamed soups in restaurants almost always have a cream or whole milk base. If you enjoy this type of soup, try our homemade versions that are made with skim milk and are equally delicious.

Vegetables and Legumes

All vegetables are acceptable until someone modifies them in the preparation. Don't be shy, ask about the preparation! Vegetables should not be prepared with egg yolk, butter, or cream sauce. The sauce is usually added at the last minute in a restaurant; you can then easily ask to have yours omitted. All fresh vegetables can be eaten to your heart's content, providing you don't add fats in the form of sauce or butter.

Legumes or beans may be included as long as they are prepared without any saturated fat. These serve as a good source of protein without saturated fat.

Salads

Salads can be made from either fruit, vegetables, chicken, or fish. Large chicken or fish salads can easily form an entire meal. Order a dressing with an oil base such as French or Italian dressing. A small amount of commercial mayonnaise is permissible because it contains very little egg yolk. If you do order mayonnaise, have it served on the side so that you will know exactly how much you are using. When cottage cheese is included in your salad, ask for the low-fat or skim-milk type if possible.

Sandwiches

You may enjoy sandwiches made with vegetables, skim milk cottage cheese, tuna, salmon, sardines, chicken, peanut butter, jam, or jelly. When ordering a sandwich, you must specify each and every time, "no butter"; when the sandwich arrives, check to see if the butter was really omitted. There is little sense in eating unwanted butter that you cannot taste and wouldn't miss if it wasn't there. If you find the bread dry, use a salad dressing type of mayonnaise in place of butter. Sliced tomatoes, cucumbers, lettuce, mustard, catsup, relish, or pickles all help dress up a sandwich without adding fat.

Meat

In a restaurant veal, lamb, or beef may be eaten if it is lean enough, but remember to remove all visible fat. Use condiments such as relishes in place of sauces and gravies that contain fat. It is preferable to order veal rather than beef in a restaurant because restaurant cuts of beef usually contain even more fat than the same cuts available at the supermarket. Save the beef for when you are at home and it can be prepared with tender loving care to minimize the fat content. If you decide to order a steak, choose only sirloin or tenderloin since these have less fat than other cuts. Rib steaks and roasts should be avoided because they are too heavily marbled with fat.

Poultry

Poultry is a good choice for lunch or dinner. It can be ordered in many different ways for variety, and makes good sandwiches, salads, or main courses. Use cranberries or condiments in place of gravy and stuffing that may be made with fat. Remove the skin, which contains the most concentrated source of fat in chicken. The meat of the chicken is a good source of protein and contains very little saturated fat. Rely on this for safe restaurant eating.

Fish

Fish, either hot or cold, answers the question of what is best to eat when dining out. There are so many varieties available that it is often hard to decide which to order. You can have your fish broiled, steamed, baked, smoked, or pickled. Ask to have it prepared without butter and to have any sauce served on the side. Moisten the fish with tartar sauce or catsup and you will never miss the butter.

If necessary, you may use a sauce sparingly. You will be amazed at how much taste can come from just a small amount and how much we overkill our taste buds by heaping large amounts of sauces on food. This is a good point to remember for any food. A small amount of cheese on a cracker tastes as good as a large amount, but the amount of fat consumed is very much different. Another example is adding sour cream or butter to a baked potato. You should learn to eat the potato without either of these additions, but if you must have some, place it on your bread plate and have a small dab on each forkful. You will be surprised at how little is necessary.

Desserts

In restaurants you should choose from Jell-O, stewed or fresh fruit, sherbets, or angel food cake without icing. You can prepare so many delicious desserts without saturated fat by following the recipes in this book that you should save your rich-tasting desserts for when you are home.

Miscellaneous

The acceptable beverages are fruit juice, vegetable juice, tea, coffee, skim milk, skim milk buttermilk, soft drinks, beer, and so on. Just avoid any beverage containing whole milk, cream, or milk substitutes.

Another product to be careful about is margarine. While certain special margarines can be used sparingly at home, the margarines used in most restaurants are not of an acceptable type and are hardly better for you than butter, so avoid them if possible.

Chinese food is generally a good choice when eating out, providing you do not order spare ribs or dishes that contain fatty pork. It is best to order dishes that contain chicken or fish, although even beef in a Chinese restaurant is usually acceptable because it is lean and served sparingly.

You may eat any kind of candy except butter toffee or candy made from regular or white chocolate. You can have hard candies, mints, jellybeans, gumdrops, and marshmallow or mint patties (without chocolate). We have some excellent and easy recipes for chocolate candy in this book so you can make your own.

Businessman's Lunch

If you often eat at the same restaurant, for example the one near your office, perhaps the owner will order some things especially for you. He may stock some skim milk, skim milk cottage cheese, fat-free soups, fat-free baked beans, flavored gelatin or unfrosted angel cake. He should certainly be able to prepare your meat, fish, or poultry without adding butter. No doubt there are many other customers who are also interested in controlling their saturated fat intake.

Dining at a Banquet or in Someone's Home

There will be times when you are a guest in someone's home or at a banquet and you do not have a choice of menu. If the food is delicious and you can't resist it, eat it and let this be your "cheat" for the month. In these situations, however, there are still ways of keeping your hard or saturated fat intake to a minimum. Whether you are served meat, fish, or poultry, you can remove the skin, trim the fat, and minimize the gravy or sauce. Remember at dessert time that most fat is in the cake icings, fillings, and in pie crusts—so eat the cake and pie filling and leave the rest. It is possible to enjoy yourself, be gracious to your hostess, and not really do too much harm by digressing from your dietary pattern.

Your day-to-day eating habits are most important for success in fat control. It is far better to go off your new way of eating on these very infrequent occasions than it is to cheat a little every day. This is very important! A once-in-a-while fling will not be handled by your body in the same way as constant, daily amounts of fat will be. With these suggestions for judicious ordering in restaurants, you can eat well, satisfy your taste buds, and still maintain your goal.

INSTANT GUIDE FOR EATING OUT

CHOOSE	AVOID
Juices	Cheese (except cottage cheese)
Clear soups	Eggs
Fruit cup	Butter or margarine
Fish	Sauces
Chicken	Creamed food
Lean meat—	Fatty meat and stews
boiled, baked, broiled	Casseroles
Cereals	Shellfish
Sandwiches	Thick soups
Plain bread and rolls	Pizza and pastas
Sherbets	Ice cream
Angel food cake	Cakes and pies
Gelatin	Pudding
Fruit	Icings and whipped toppings

Chapter 12 • Hors d'oeuvres and Lunch

Because we think of lunch as a quick meal, we often turn to food very high on our unwanted list: eggs, luncheon meat, French toast, or any of a large number of instant meals found in supermarket freezers that are rich in saturated fat. For this reason, we have taken particular care to offer practical suggestions for replacing these harmful lunches with healthy, but equally simple, alternatives.

In this section the hors d'oeuvres are grouped with luncheon meals because, with slight changes in quantity, the same food can do for either. For example, pizza, meatballs, or onion quiche can be either an appetizer or lunch depending on the amount served and what accompanies it.

A good example of an hors d'oeuvre that has grown up into a luncheon dish is the Hot Hamburger Canape. Try this idea using a submarine roll or French bread as a base.

For a somewhat more elegant lunch, the crepes are excellent, even though they take a little extra time. They are also excellent for a late evening party meal or as the first course for company. We have never had any leftovers no matter when they were served.

Scan the recipes to find more suggestions for healthier lunches. Stay away from the frozen food packages that line the shelves of our supermarkets. Eating these commercially prepared foods is the best way to load up on unwanted saturated fats. Especially harmful are the fried foods, pot pies, and T.V. dinners because they contain shortening or lard. Prepare your own using oil; they are much tastier, more healthful, and cheaper.

Sandwiches

There are so many possibilities in sandwich preparations that your imagination can take you far if you follow the basic guidelines. These can range from open-faced sandwiches for parties to the daily needs of children's lunch boxes. Your new approach to eating carries just a few new rules. A salad dressing type of mayonnaise must be used in place of butter. This is such a satisfying substitute that you won't even taste the difference. Never use prepared or canned meat—

you have no way of knowing what the fat content is and it is usually high. Instead of the cream cheese variety of fillings available in the dairy case, try our substitutions made with skim milk cottage cheese.

When buying peanut butter for those ever-popular peanut butter and jelly sandwiches, remember that "hydrogenated" is taboo, but "homogenized" is allowed. To be really economical and sure of the oil content, learn how to make your own peanut butter. (See page 63.)

Because egg yolks are very rich in cholesterol, chopped egg sandwiches must be modified if you are to eat them. To make chopped egg sandwich filling, use two whites to one yolk and add some chopped olives, celery, or chives. Note that much less salad dressing will be needed because it is the yolk that is dry. You will be surprised how little you will miss the yolk, and think of how much fat and cholesterol you will avoid.

Snacks

Potato chips, buttered popcorn, fried onion rings, and many commercial snacks are great offenders and have little nutritional value. As a substitute for these kinds of snacks, try our recipe for Nuts and Bolts. Vary the cereals and spices. Your local supermarket has seasonings such as barbecue- or pizza-flavored granules that can give a variety of flavors to these snacks.

Nuts

All types of nuts are acceptable, but if you buy the roasted type make sure that they are dry roasted with no saturated fat added. Try mixing shelled nuts and raisins. Try almonds in this very nutritious snack.

Dips

Have fun experimenting with different dips using our basic recipe instead of commercial sour cream, which is forbidden. For party serving, cut the tops off green or red peppers, hollow, and use them as festive containers. They will give added flavor and color. No one will miss potato chips with a dip when you can serve melba toast or an attractive plate of raw vegetables for the same purpose. These can include radish roses, raw cauliflower flowerets, carrot and celery sticks, and cucumber slices.

Snacks and hors d'oeuvres are potential sources of unhealthy foods, but need not be so. Instead of buying commercially prepared snacks containing excess fat as a last-minute thought, plan ahead so you can make your own delicious and nutritious appetizers.

NUTS AND BOLTS

Combine:
⅓ cup oil
1 tablespoon Worcestershire sauce
garlic salt to taste
2 cups Cheerios
2 cups Corn Chex or Wheat Chex
1 cup shelled mixed nuts
2 cups thin pretzel sticks

Place in a large, flat pan and put in a 250° oven for 45 minutes, stirring every 15 minutes. Cool on absorbent towels. Store in an airtight container. For variety, vary the cereals and spices.

MARINATED VEGETABLES

This is an attractive and easy hors d'oeuvre to prepare.

Drain:
1 can artichoke hearts

Combine with:
cherry tomatoes
raw mushroom caps

Marinate these vegetables in your favorite Italian dressing or use the Italian dressing given in a later section.

STUFFED TOMATO HORS D'OEUVRES

Slit cherry tomatoes into quarters, cutting three-quarters of the way down and spread open. Fill with a half teaspoon of any of the following:

salmon salad
chicken salad
tuna salad
seasoned cottage cheese

Serve cold.

MOCK SHRIMP COCKTAIL

Boil in 1 quart
of water for 15
minutes:
1 small onion, quartered
1 teaspoon salt
1 bay leaf
6 whole black peppercorns
½ teaspoon sugar

Add: **1 pound of halibut (any firm white fish may be substituted) cut into shrimp-sized pieces**

Cook until firm. Remove from water and chill. Serve with cocktail sauce.

CHOPPED CHICKEN LIVER

Sauté until golden: **3 tablespoons oil**
1 large onion, chopped
salt and pepper to taste
3 generous shakes of paprika

Add: **1 teaspoon instant chicken soup powder**
1 pound well-cleaned chicken livers (make sure all green veins are cut away)

Simmer covered for 10 minutes or until livers are cooked.

Put livers through
meat grinder with: **2 hard-boiled eggs less 1 yolk**

Mix together and taste; add more seasoning if necessary. If mixture is too dry, add a little boiling water.

Chopped liver makes a lovely paté for a party, and is also delicious in sandwiches or as a salad base.

MOCK CHOPPED LIVER

Sauté until golden: **1 large onion, chopped**
2 tablespoons oil
salt and pepper to taste
dash of paprika

Put the following through the fine blade of a meat grinder or chop until fine:

                      cooked onion mixture
1 pound cooked green string beans (well drained)
3 hard-boiled eggs (less 1 yolk)
½ teaspoon powdered chicken soup

Serve cold as an hors d'oeuvre or use as a base for a salad.

BASIC CREAM,
OR WHITE SAUCE

Heat slightly over
medium heat: **2 tablespoons oil**

Add and stir until
pale yellow: **2 tablespoons flour**

Add: **1 cup skim milk**

Add the milk all at once, stirring constantly until the mixture is smooth and comes to a boil.

Season with: ¼ teaspoon salt
                     dash of pepper

This makes a medium sauce. For a thicker sauce, use 3 tablespoons oil and 3 tablespoons flour and prepare as above. For a thinner sauce, use 1 tablespoon oil and 1 tablespoon flour and prepare as above.

This sauce can be the base for a variety of dishes by adding approximately equal amounts of solids to the sauce. Try some of the following:

> chunks of turkey
> chunks of chicken
> chunks of white tuna (drained)
> cooked fish
> sautéed mushrooms

For flavor and   canned peas
color add: pimentos cut in pieces

Serve in toast baskets or over plain toast.

CREAM OF MUSHROOM SOUP (CONDENSED)

Use preceding basic cream sauce and add:

> ½ cup finely chopped mushrooms, sautéed in
> 1 teaspoon oil

This can be used in place of canned cream of mushroom soup in all your own recipes.

COTTAGE CHEESE MOCK SOUR CREAM

A delicious, commercial type of "sour cream" can be made from low-fat cottage cheese. The consistency of the cheese varies from brand to brand so these instructions must be general. If the cheese is very moist, use less milk, and if it is very dry, a little more milk may be necessary.

Blend: ½ pound cottage cheese
               ⅓ to ½ cup skim milk or skim milk buttermilk

Keep blending until the desired consistency is reached. It will make about 1½ cups "sour cream." This "cream" will keep refrigerated as long as the cheese would have.

For a "cream cheese," proceed as above, using much less liquid.

HERRING IN "SOUR CREAM"

Drain: 1 12-ounce jar of "herring tidbits in wine sauce"

Cut the larger pieces in half and add:	¼ **of an apple peeled and thinly sliced** ¼ **of an orange (peel and fruit) very finely sliced** ¼ **cup raisins** ½ **cup "sour cream" (see recipe) or natural-flavored skim milk yogurt**

Refrigerate for 12 hours before serving.

This may sound like an unusual combination, but in order not to be embarrassed by running short, make sure you have plenty on hand.

RAW VEGETABLE DIP FOR WEIGHT WATCHERS

To:	1 **cup "sour cream" (see recipe)**
Add very finely chopped:	**3 scallions or shallots** ¼ **medium green pepper** **a few sprigs of parsley** **6-8 radishes** ¼ **cucumber** 1 **very firm tomato** 1 **small carrot** ¼ **teaspoon salt** **liberal amount fresh ground pepper**
Serve well chilled and for dippers use:	**cucumber slices** **green pepper strips** **carrot curls** **celery chunks**

"CREAM CHEESE" SPREADS

To one-half cup "sour cream" (see recipe) made very thick, add any of the following:

2 tablespoons crushed pineapple

or

2 tablespoons mixed sweet relish

or

2 tablespoons well-drained diced pimento

or

2 tablespoons chopped stuffed olives

"SOUR CREAM" DIPS

To one cup "sour cream" (see recipe) add any of the following (or invent your own):

anchovies finely minced

or

chopped black olives

or

chopped stuffed olives

or

dehydrated onion soup mix

or

dehydrated mixed vegetables

Serve surrounded by melba toast, thinly sliced pumpernickle, or raw vegetables.

VEGETABLE LUNCH BOWL

Cut into bite-size pieces:

cucumber
green pepper
tomatoes
radishes
scallions

Cover with "sour cream" (see recipe) and add:

salt
fresh ground pepper

Serve cold with melba toast. If you prefer, this is equally as good with natural-flavored skim milk yogurt.

HORS D'OEUVRE MEATBALLS

Combine and roll into small balls:

2 pounds lean ground beef
1 egg white
1 teaspoon salt
⅓ cup bread crumbs

Combine the following in a large pot:

1 11-ounce jar of grape or apple jelly
1 11-ounce jar of chili sauce
1 teaspoon lemon juice

Bring to a boil. Add the meatballs to sauce and cook covered for 20 minutes, then uncovered for another 20 minutes. Serve hot.

BAKED STUFFED MUSHROOM CAPS

Wash, pat dry, sprinkle with salt, and set aside:

18 to 24 large mushroom caps

Heat in skillet:

2 tablespoons oil

Add and cook for 2 minutes or until tender:

4 tablespoons finely chopped scallions

Stir in and toss for about 10 seconds:

1½ cups crabmeat

Put this mixture in a bowl, add:	**1 cup white sauce (see recipe), medium thickness** **¼ teaspoon lemon juice** **salt and white pepper**

Arrange the caps in a shallow, greased baking dish. Spoon filling in mushroom caps. Bake in the upper part of the oven at 350° for 10-15 minutes. Serve on a heated platter.

HOT HAMBURGER CANAPES

Cut into bite-size pieces—rounds, squares or triangles:

4 slices of rye or kimmel bread

Spread ⅛-inch thick with:	**lean raw ground beef** **salt**

In the center of each piece place a dab of:

catsup

Broil 3 to 4 minutes until brown. Serve hot and make sure you have plenty.

BOUCHÉES OR CREAM PUFF SHELLS

Prepare cream puff shell dough as described in chapter 19 making very small puffs and using about one-half teaspoonful of dough. When the shells are cool, cut open on one side near the top, and fill with creamed chicken, tuna, or mushrooms. Just before serving, heat in a 350° oven for 5-6 minutes.

Unfilled puff shells can be prepared in advance and refrigerated for a day or two until needed. They can also be frozen and then defrosted and filled.

GARLIC "SPARERIBS"

Stir together:	**1 tablespoon oil** **1 tablespoon soy sauce** **1 tablespoon white sugar** **1 tablespoon brown sugar** **1 clove garlic crushed (garlic salt or powder may be substituted)** **¼ cup water**
Place:	**½ pound well-trimmed veal rib bones**

in the sauce. Bake for one hour in 450° oven, basting often. Add more water if the sauce thickens too much.

QUICK PIZZA

Place on a cookie sheet:	**6 English muffin halves**
Cover with:	**marinara or meatless spaghetti sauce**
Top with any or all of the following:	**green pepper slices**
	anchovy fillets
	mushroom slices
	small stuffed olives
	imitation bacon bits
	small amount of grated skim milk mozzarella cheese

Bake in a 450° oven for about 10 minutes until cheese is melted. Serve hot.

These may be prepared in advance and refrigerated until baking time.

TOAST BASKETS

Use one slice of bread for each basket. Trim the crust leaving a square of bread. Make a cut from each corner halfway to the center.

Brush the bread lightly with oil, and place each slice in a muffin tin, overlapping each cut corner to make a pinwheel-shaped cup. Press the bread against the sides to squeeze the overlapping sections together.

Bake in a 350° oven for 5 minutes or until golden. These may be made early in the day and are excellent to hold creamed fillings, sautéed chicken livers, and so on.

MUSHROOMS AND ONIONS IN BASKETS

Sauté until golden:	**3 large onions halved and then sliced ¼ inch thick**
Add:	**½ pound fresh mushrooms sliced**
	1 stalk celery thinly sliced
	1 red or green sweet pepper thinly sliced
	salt, pepper, and paprika to taste

Cover and simmer until vegetables are crisply tender.

Add:	**2 tomatoes cut in eighths**

Cook an additional 5 minutes and serve on toast or in toast baskets.

ONION QUICHE

Prepare:	**1 9-inch "no-roll" pie shell (see chapter 19)**

and bake in a 400° oven for 10 minutes.

Heat in a skillet:	**2 tablespoons oil**

Add: **4 chopped onions**

Cook uncovered over very low heat until tender, about 1 hour.

Stir in: **1 tablespoon flour**

In mixing bowl
beat: **1 egg**

Add: **½ cup skim milk**
                        ½ teaspoon salt
                        dash pepper

Spread the cooked onions over the dough and over that sprinkle:

                        1 ounce grated skim milk cheese
                        ¼ cup imitation bacon bits such as Bac*Os

Spoon the egg mixture evenly over this. Bake in a 375° oven 35-40 minutes or until the top is golden brown.

This pie, served with a salad and garlic bread, makes an appetizing late night supper or an afternoon luncheon. Serve with a chilled white wine.

This recipe can also be used to make appetizers. Prepare tart shells and proceed as above, but bake for only 20 minutes. These can be frozen and reheated, but we suggest that you defrost them thoroughly before reheating.

NOODLE PUDDING

Boil in salted water and drain:

                        1 8-ounce package of medium-sized noodles

Mix together: **½ cup oil**
                        ½ cup sugar
                        2 egg yolks
                        1 teaspoon vanilla
                        ¾ cup skim milk
                        2 tablespoons skim milk powder
                        rind and juice of ½ lemon
                        4 apples peeled and diced
                        ½ cup raisins
                        6 dried apricot halves finely cut (optional)
                        ½ teaspoon salt
                        ½ teaspoon cinnamon

Add cooked noodles.

Beat until stiff: **3 egg whites**

Fold into noodle mixture.

Spoon into lightly oiled 9 x 12 inch baking dish. Sprinkle topping over noodle mixture. Bake in 350° oven for one hour. Serve hot or cold with a dab of "sour cream."

Topping

Blend together:
- ½ teaspoon cinnamon
- 2 tablespoons brown sugar
- ¼ cup dry cereal rolled into crumbs (corn flakes or Grape Nut Flakes)
- 2 teaspoons oil

RIBBON PARTY SANDWICHES

Prepare filling as for salads:
- **chopped egg (use 1 yolk to two whites)**
- **salmon salad**
- **tuna salad**
- **chicken salad**
- **sardines**

Use thinly sliced bread with crusts left on (whole wheat or white).

Spread four slices of bread with salad dressing and then three of them with any combination of the above filling. On top of each filling place one of the following:

- **thinly sliced cucumber**
- **thinly sliced tomato**
- **sliced olives**
- **sliced pimentos**
- **sliced gherkins**

Cover with the fourth slice of bread. Then wrap tightly in waxed paper or plastic wrap, cover with a damp towel, and refrigerate for a few hours or overnight. Before serving, trim crusts using a sharp knife and slice half-inch thick strips or triangles. Arrange on platters garnished with olives, gherkins, and radish roses.

Leftover ribbon sandwiches, when broiled filling side up, make a delicious snack. If you omit or remove the tomato or cucumber, you can freeze them and defrost by broiling—a perfect last-minute lunch or late-night snack.

Peanut butter, jelly, and banana are popular for a young child's birthday party. For an adult crowd, ribbon sandwiches made from chopped liver, sliced turkey, or chicken salad on rye or whole wheat add an unusual touch to a cold buffet.

TUNA ANTIPASTO

Combine in a bowl:
- ¼ cup catsup
- ¼ cup piccalilli tomato relish (hot if desired)
- ½ cup sliced or diced carrots (cooked or canned)
- ½ cup sliced celery, cooked
- ¼ cup sliced olives

⅓ cup sliced sweet gherkins
garlic to taste
2 tablespoons oil

Add: 1 can tuna drained and flaked

Allow to marinate for two or three days. This will keep in a glass jar in the refrigerator for three to four weeks—if your family doesn't eat it first.

TUNA PINEAPPLE SALAD

Combine: 1 7-ounce can tuna
½ cup stuffed green olives, chopped
½ cup raw carrots, grated
1 tablespoon grated onion
¼ cup mayonnaise (salad dressing type)

Mix thoroughly.

Using: 8 slices of pineapple (well drained)

make "sandwiches" of tuna mixture and arrange on salad plates garnished with tomatoes and green peppers.

TUNA BENEDICT

Drain, rinse, break into large pieces, and set aside:

1 7-ounce can of tuna

Heat in a
saucepan: 2 tablespoons oil

Sprinkle in: 2 tablespoons flour
¾ teaspoon salt
⅛ teaspoon pepper

Remove from heat and add:

2 cups skim milk

Return to moderate heat and cook, stirring constantly, until sauce is thickened and smooth.

Add and heat   2 tablespoons chopped parsley
thoroughly: 1 tablespoon grated onion
                 dash of Tabasco sauce
                 tuna pieces

Toast: 3 English muffins

Top each muffin half with a part of the tuna mixture.

BROILED TUNA-CHEESE SANDWICHES

Combine: 1 7-ounce can of tuna, drained
1½ teaspoons prepared mustard

¼ teaspoon Worcestershire sauce
3 tablespoons mayonnaise (salad dressing type)
1½ teaspoons grated onion
2 tablespoons chopped green pepper

Divide this mixture and put it on:

3 open hamburger buns (6 halves)

Top with: tomato slices

Mix together and spread sparingly over tomatoes:

2 tablespoons mayonnaise (salad dressing type)
2 tablespoons grated skim milk cheese

Broil 2 or 3 minutes and serve at once.

FRENCH TOAST

With a fork
beat together: 2 egg whites
1 egg yolk
3 tablespoons skim milk
1 tablespoon instant skim milk powder
dash of salt

Soak in the egg mixture:

3 slices of bread

In lightly oiled frying pan, fry on both sides until brown. Serve with jam, maple syrup, or cinnamon and sugar.

CHEESE MANICOTTI

Blintz or Crêpe Dough

Combine and stir until the consistency of a very light cream:

2 eggs
¾ cup flour
½ teaspoon salt
1 cup skim milk

Heat and very lightly oil a six-inch frying pan. Pour about 3 tablespoons of batter into the hot pan and tip to spread evenly. When brown underneath, turn out on counter. Repeat. If first pancake seems too thick, add a little more milk to batter and continue. Makes about 12 crêpes.

Filling

Combine: 1 pound cottage cheese
¼ pound skim milk mozzarella cheese, diced
¼ cup Italian seasoned bread crumbs
2 tablespoons chopped parsley
1 egg
¼ teaspoon salt

Place spoonfuls of filling on center of crêpes. Fold into squares and arrange in lightly oiled baking dish. Fills 12 manicotti.

Cover with: **¾ cup marinara or meatless spaghetti sauce**

Bake in 350° oven for 30 minutes. There are pasta manicotti shells available if you prefer. Parboil according to instructions on the box and fill with above mixture. Both types may be filled and frozen. Bake just before serving. Served with a salad, it makes a filling meatless meal.

COTTAGE CHEESE SANDWICH

Sieve or blend until of spreading consistency:

8 ounces cottage cheese

Add: **¼ teaspoon cinnamon**
1 teaspoon sugar
raisins if desired

Make 6 sandwiches using:

white or raisin bread

Beat together
until frothy: **3 egg whites**
1 egg yolk
3 tablespoons skim milk
pinch of salt

Dip the sandwiches in the egg mixture and fry until brown in:

2 tablespoons oil

Serve topped with fresh fruit, fruit sauce, or maple syrup.

CHEESE DELIGHTS (BAGEL)

Filling

Beat until smooth
and set aside: **1 pound cottage cheese**
1 egg
¼ teaspoon salt
2 tablespoons sugar
1 teaspoon vanilla

Dough

In a large bowl,
combine: **2 cups flour**
2 teaspoons baking powder
⅛ teaspoon salt
½ cup sugar

Make a well
and add: **1 egg**
½ cup oil
½ cup skim milk

Mix thoroughly handling as little as possible (this is a very soft dough). Divide dough into 2 parts. On floured board, roll each part into a rectangular shape approximately 7 x 14 inches. Spread half the filling on the dough and roll as for a jelly roll. Cut into 1½ inch slices. Place cut side down on a lightly oiled cookie sheet and pinch upper ends together. Repeat with the remainder of the dough and filling. Bake in 350° oven about 30 minutes or until golden. Serve warm with "sour cream" (see recipe) and strawberries or with fruit-flavored yogurt. These are very handy to have in the freezer to pop into your oven for instant use.

CHEESE PIE

Filling

Combine with electric mixer and set aside:	2 pounds cottage cheese
	2 eggs less 1 yolk
	¼ cup sugar
	¼ teaspoon salt
	¼ teaspoon cinnamon
	⅓ cup seedless raisins
	skim milk (if needed to make the mixture spreadable)

Batter

Combine:	½ cup oil
	1 cup sugar
	2 eggs
Then add, stirring until well blended:	2 cups all-purpose flour
	3½ teaspoons baking powder
	¼ teaspoon salt
	1 cup skim milk
	1 teaspoon vanilla

Place the batter into two lightly oiled 9-inch pie plates, building up the sides. Drop the cheese mixture by the tablespoon evenly on the batter. Sprinkle the top with a mixture of:

cinnamon and sugar

Bake in 350° oven for 45 minutes or until brown. Serve hot with "sour cream" (see recipe) and a fruit sauce.

STUFFED CRÊPES

Crêpes

The following recipe is made in an electric blender because it is so quick. (If you do not have one, use an electric mixer—beat the eggs until light and then, beating constantly, add alternately flour and salt, milk and oil.) Crêpe batter should be made and refrigerated for at least 2 hours before being used. This insures a thin, tender crêpe.

Place into the blender jar:	1 cup cold skim milk
	2 eggs
	¼ teaspoon salt

Then add: **1 cup sifted all-purpose flour**
2 tablespoons oil

Cover and blend for 1 minute at high speed. Refrigerate covered for at least 2 hours. The batter should be like a very light cream. If after your first crêpe the batter seems too heavy, beat a bit of water into it, a spoonful at a time.

Heat a 6-inch skillet. Grease it with:

a few drops of oil

Add a small quantity of batter (about ¼ cup). Tip the skillet and let the batter spread over the bottom. Cook the pancake over moderate heat. When it is brown underneath, reverse it and lightly brown the other side. Use a few drops of oil when needed. Slide the crêpes onto a plate. They may be made several hours in advance and reheated. This recipe makes 18 crêpes. The crêpes can be separated by waxed paper, wrapped carefully, and frozen. If you do this, remember to thaw them well before filling.

Filling for Crêpes

Prepare: **3 cups white sauce (see recipe)**

Season with: **salt**
pepper
garlic salt

Set aside one cup.

To the remaining **2 cups chopped cooked chicken (crabmeat or tuna)**
2 cups, add: **½ cup cooked mushrooms**
½ cup chopped pimentos

Place about 2 tablespoons of filling on each crêpe. Fold and tuck ends under. Place in a lightly oiled baking dish.

To the sauce that you set aside, add:

2 tablespoons grated skim milk cheese

Cover the crêpes with the sauce. Bake in a 350° oven 10 minutes.

CRÊPE MOUNDS

For an interesting entree or main course dish, crêpes can be piled flat in a shallow baking dish with filling between each, and then covered with a well-seasoned white sauce (see recipe). They can also be spread with minced cooked veal or chicken to which cooked vegetables such as eggplant, mushrooms, or spinach have been added, and then covered with a tomato sauce.

These crêpe dishes can be made ready for the oven in the morning and heated up at dinner time.

Chapter 13 • Soups

Starting a meal with a good soup often means that you will forego that extra helping of meat. This is a far better way to feel satisfied after a meal and feeling satisfied is the key to successful eating. It is even better to enjoy the soup and main dish knowing that you have properly limited your meat and fat to a healthy level.

The ability to prepare a good soup is a most rewarding talent. Soups are nutritious, contain large quantities of protein and vitamins, and fill a special need in our diets. After mastering the basic rules for preparing fat-free soups, you can use your ingenuity to combine ingredients.

Stock

The trick to making many soups is to have a basic stock. Such a recipe is included in this section. This stock must be prepared beforehand and placed in the refrigerator to cool. Then the layer of fat that forms on the top must be removed before the stock is used.

A quick stock may be made from bouillon cubes, canned clear soup, or dried bases. Short ribs (or flanken) are too marbled with fat to be used in preparing a soup base, but you can use knuckle bones. Scrape out all the marrow you can from the bones before cooking. If you want to add meat, use very lean stewing beef.

Stocks can be prepared beforehand and then stored in your freezer. Prepared by any of these methods, the stock is then available as the basic ingredient for a number of soups found in this recipe section, or for any of your family's favorites.

Creamed Soups

Creamed soups must be homemade to be certain that they contain no cream or whole milk. You may follow your own recipes, using skim milk in place of whole milk or cream, and adding a few spoons of oil in place of butter. For a richer soup, add more skim milk powder. Remember, any creamed soup will be ruined by boiling, so be sure to heat just to the boiling point. To reheat, place the soup in the top of a double boiler over hot water.

Instant Mixes

Instant soup mixes are one of the few convenience foods that you can buy with safety. The basic flavors are chicken, beef, onion, and mushroom. These are very handy since they have many uses other than preparation of stock. They can be used as a fast, hot, pick-me-up drink in the middle of the day when you want a change from tea or coffee. A teaspoonful of instant soup mix will also enhance the flavor of stews, gravies, vegetables, instant potatoes, or rice.

Flavor

Learn to use herbs and seasonings to delight your family with unusually flavored soup sensations. Chervil, thyme, basil, and tarragon are spices that will enhance any soup. Should your soup be too salty, add a potato cut into eighths, cook until the potato is tender, remove the potato and discard. The potato will have absorbed the excess salt.

Many soups can be frozen. Remember to leave room at the top of the container since the soup will expand when it freezes.

Canned Soup

If you use canned soups, check the label carefully for unwanted ingredients. Using canned soups or vegetables as a base, you can make your own interesting combinations. For example:

—to green pea soup add ¼ cup sherry and croutons
—to onion soup or consommé add 2 tablespoons sherry
—to tomato soup add ½ cup cooked rice
—to chicken broth add 2 tablespoons white wine
—combine a can of tomato soup and a can of pea soup

Garnishes

A plain soup or broth can always be made more appealing by adding an attractive garnish or accompaniment. Try some of the following:

—croutons or toast points in pea or tomato soup
—soup dumplings or matzo balls in chicken soup or bouillon
—very thin orange slices in a creamed soup
—nutmeg or cloves sprinkled on a cream or vegetable soup
—chopped chives in vichyssoise
—caraway seeds sprinkled on vegetable soup
—toasted almonds sprinkled on a creamed soup or bouillon

A hearty soup, such as seafood chowder, vegetable soup, or French onion soup, is a filling and satisfying meal in itself. It need only be accompanied by hot bread or rolls and a salad. A lighter soup, such as a creamed soup, can be used as a luncheon dish or as the first course for dinner. Try to remember to serve soup on a night that you are serving beef, and allow the soup to help fill you up so that you will eat less of the red meat.

BASIC SOUP STOCK

Soup stock must be made the day before you need it so that the stock can be chilled and the cake of fat that comes to the top can be easily removed. If you think you can accomplish the same thing by skipping the stock procedure and skimming after the soup has been cooked, forget it; the vegetables will act as sponges and absorb the fat. This fat can never be removed then. We have found that knee bones make an excellent stock and they are inexpensive. To prepare bones, scoop out and discard any marrow that may be present. If you must use meat, buy the leanest you can find (never flank or short ribs), trim all visible fat and proceed.

In a large soup pot, combine:	2 quarts cold water knee bones lean meat cubed (if desired) 1 bay leaf 1 tablespoon salt 6 peppercorns 1 onion sliced 2 carrots

Cover and simmer slowly for 2 hours. Remove meat and bones, strain soup, and chill.

QUICK CHICKEN SOUP

In a saucepan combine:	1 carrot sliced 1 onion quartered 1 stalk of celery ¼ teaspoon dried dill a few shakes of ginger ½ teaspoon salt 4 cups cold water 4 teaspoons chicken soup powder

Boil together, partially covered, until vegetables are tender. Serve with "5-minute" rice.

CHICKEN SOUP AND MATZO BALLS

Place in a large pot and cover with cold water:

> **1 3-pound boiling fowl (whole or cut up, skin removed)**

When water is boiling rapidly, remove the scum and fat that comes to the top and then add:

> **4 large carrots**
> **3 stalks celery with leaves**
> **1 large onion**
> **½ bunch fresh dill (or 1 tablespoon dried dill)**
> **1 small parsnip (optional)**
> **2 tablespoons salt**
> **1-inch piece of dried ginger root (or ¼ teaspoon dried ginger)**
> **¼ teaspoon sugar**

Continue cooking partially covered until chicken is tender. Strain and then chill so you can easily remove any fat that comes to the top. Serve with matzo balls. Any leftover chicken may be used in creamed dishes, in sandwiches, or in many other chicken recipes.

Matzo Balls

Beat until stiff: **1 egg white**

Add the following and stir until well blended: **1 beaten yolk**
salt
pepper
¼ cup matzo meal

Refrigerate the mixture for about 20 minutes for ease in rolling. Form small balls using moderate pressure. Drop into boiling, salted water. Use a large pot because the balls will double in size. Boil covered for 45 minutes. They may then be transferred to the soup. Makes about 10 balls.

This light, fluffy ball is delicious when served with a beef stew, and, surprisingly, it freezes beautifully.

BEAN AND BARLEY SOUP

Place in a large soup pot: **2 quarts stock**
4 carrots cut up
2 stalks diced celery
1 diced onion
½ cup barley
¾ cup dried lima beans
salt and pepper to taste

Allow to simmer for 2 hours partially covered, stirring from time to time to prevent the barley from sticking.

PURÉE OF PEA SOUP

In approximately:	**2 quarts of stock**
simmer covered until very tender:	**3 large carrots cut in pieces**
	1 small onion, quartered
	2 stalks celery
	1 cup dried split green peas
	salt and pepper to taste

Simmer partially covered for about 2 hours until the vegetables are very tender. Strain soup through a food mill. Serve hot with croutons.

ONION SOUP

In a covered saucepan, sauté until golden:	**6 onions thinly sliced**
	2 tablespoons oil
Blend in thoroughly:	**1 tablespoon flour**
Add:	**4 cups beef consommé**
	1½ tablespoons dry white wine
	salt and pepper to taste
	garlic salt to taste

Simmer partially covered for ½ to 1 hour. Pour the soup into ovenproof soup bowls.

Then add:	**small amount grated mozzarella cheese**
Cover with:	**toast rounds**

Bake covered for 20 minutes at 350°. Then broil for 1 to 2 minutes. Serves 4 to 5 people.

Toast Rounds

Bake slices of French bread in 325° oven for ½ hour.

Sprinkle with:	**oil**
halfway through baking.	

QUICK ONION SOUP

A very fast version.

Sauté until golden, about 15 minutes:	**2 large, sliced onions in**
	2 tablespoons oil
	salt and pepper to taste
Add:	**1 teaspoon flour**
stirring constantly.	

Dissolve:
2 teaspoons instant chicken or beef broth in
2 cups water
a shake of garlic salt

Add to onions and simmer for five minutes.

Brush two slices of white bread with oil and toast lightly. Cover with a little grated mozzarella cheese and continue toasting.

Serve soup with toast floating on top.

VEGETABLE SOUP

Place in a large soup pot:
2 quarts stock
4 carrots, diced
2 stalks celery, diced
1 onion, chopped
1 can tomato soup
pieces of lean soup meal or knee gristle (optional)

Add 4 cups of any or all of the following:
peas
cut green beans
corn (cut off the cob)
cauliflower flowerettes
any other available vegetables, cut into small pieces

Then add:
4 teaspoons salt
pepper
¼ teaspoon oregano
½ bunch dried dill (tied together with white thread for easy removal)
¼ cup washed barley
¼ cup dried lima beans

Allow to simmer partially covered about two hours, stirring frequently. Taste and add more salt if necessary.

SWEET AND PUNGENT CABBAGE SOUP

To 2 quarts defatted soup stock add:
1 can whole tomatoes cubed (19 ounces)
1 can tomato juice (28 ounces)
1 small cabbage, diced
1 onion, diced
1 cup small cubes of very lean beef (optional)
⅛ cup lima beans
juice of one-half lemon
4 tablespoons brown sugar
salt and pepper to taste

Simmer partially covered for about 3 hours. Taste, adjust seasonings, and continue to simmer for another hour.

MEATLESS POTATO SOUP

Boil together partially covered until vegetables are tender:

> 1 small onion, chopped
> 1 stalk celery, diced
> 1 cup carrots, diced
> 1½ cups potatoes, diced
> 1 teaspoon salt
> 5 cups water

In a frying pan brown well:

> 2 tablespoons oil
> 2 tablespoons flour

Then add about 1 cup of the water from the vegetables to the flour mixture. Stir until well blended and return to vegetables. Heat slowly to the boiling point and add:

> ⅓ to ½ cup skim milk powder dissolved in
> ½ cup water

Taste, and add more salt or water if necessary. Serve at once. Do not allow to boil.

This is the basic way to prepare any meatless vegetable soup. Any cooked or canned vegetables may be added or substituted.

CREAM OF MUSHROOM SOUP

Sauté and set aside:

> ½ pound finely cut mushrooms in
> 1 tablespoon oil

Cook together until bubbly and golden:

> 2 tablespoons flour
> 2 tablespoons oil

Add all at once a mixture of:

> 1 cup skim milk powder
> 4 cups water

Cook over low heat until just before the boiling point.

Add:

> 4 teaspoons condensed chicken soup powder
> salt and pepper to taste

Add the reserved mushrooms and liquid. These may be put through a blender or the finest blade of a food chopper if desired.

NEW ENGLAND CLAM CHOWDER

Cook until just tender and reserve liquid:

> 2 medium diced potatoes
> 1 thinly sliced carrot
> 1 teaspoon salt

In a 2-quart saucepan combine:

> reserved liquid with water added to make 2½ cups of liquid
> 1 cup instant skim milk powder

1 10½-ounce can of minced clams undrained
2 tablespoons oil

Cook over low heat for ten minutes.

Add: drained cooked carrots and potatoes
4 scallions, chopped
1 tablespoon chopped parsley
salt and pepper to taste

Simmer 10 minutes longer.

CREAM OF VEGETABLE SOUP

This soup can be made with many different vegetables.

Sauté:	1 tablespoon oil 1 onion, chopped
Purée and set aside:	browned onion 1½ cups cooked vegetable (broccoli, corn, carrots)
Heat in a saucepan:	2 tablespoons oil
Blend in:	2 tablespoons flour
Add:	1 10-ounce can consommé (or your own stock)

Stir until smooth and thick.

Combine and then add:	¾ cup skim milk powder 2 cups water

Bring to a boil, reduce heat, and simmer for 5 minutes.

Add:	vegetable purée salt and pepper to taste nutmeg (optional)

Keep hot until time to serve, but *do not boil*. Garnish with parsley, chives, or a few sliced vegetables.

FRENCH-CANADIAN FISH CHOWDER

Cook partially covered over low heat for 1 hour:	1 can tomatoes (whole—14 ounces) 1 can tomato juice (19 ounces) 2 large Spanish onions, sliced 5 medium sliced carrots ½ teaspoon sugar 1 teaspoon salt fresh ground pepper
Add 3½ pounds of any combination of the following:	salmon, haddock, halibut scallops, lobster, shrimp, canned baby clams (cut in bite-size pieces) 2 tablespoons oil

Cook slowly ¾ hour.

Just before serving add:

> 1 can cooked, whole, small, peeled potatoes

Serve from a tureen at the table with garlic bread, and you have a delectable meal. This chowder freezes very well. If freezing, cook fish only 15 minutes since it tends to break up when reheated, and leave out potatoes until just before serving.

BAYOU FISH CHOWDER

Heat in a large, heavy pot:

> 3 tablespoons oil

Add:

> 2 leeks, white part only, sliced thin
> 2 medium carrots, sliced
> 1 clove garlic, crushed

Cook, gently stirring, for 3 minutes.

Add:

> 1 pound haddock cut in pieces
> 2 cups peeled, chopped tomatoes
> 1 green pepper, sliced
> 1 box mushrooms, sliced
> 1 small bay leaf
> ⅛ teaspoon thyme
> 1½ teaspoons salt
> ¼ teaspoon pepper
> 2 cups water
> ¼ cup chopped parsley

Heat until boiling. Turn down heat and simmer for 10 minutes.

Add:

> 1 tablespoon lemon juice
> ½ pound scallops, cut in half

Simmer 5 minutes longer, or until scallops are tender. Sprinkle with parsley and serve.

FISH AND CORN CHOWDER

Heat over low heat:

> 1 16-ounce can creamed corn
> 2 cups water
> 3 teaspoons instant chicken soup powder
> 1 cup cooked fish pieces
>   (any type of leftover or precooked fish fillets)
> salt and pepper to taste
> 1 teaspoon freshly snipped parsley

Serve hot with crackers.

VICHYSSOISE

This soup served hot becomes "cream" of potato soup.

Split lengthwise and chop, using white parts only:

3 or 4 leeks

Heat in a heavy saucepan:

¼ cup oil

and cook leeks gently until soft but not brown.

Add:
4 thinly sliced potatoes
3 cups chicken stock
2 cups water
1½ teaspoons salt

Bring to a boil, reduce heat, and cook partially covered 35 minutes or until potatoes are very soft. Strain through fine sieve or put into blender, and reduce to a purée. Heat purée and bring to a boil again. Reduce heat and then add:

1 cup skim milk powder mixed with 1 cup water

Do not allow to boil after milk has been added. Serve either hot or cold. Garnish with chopped chives.

GAZPACHO

This is a refreshing hot-weather soup. It is made of raw vegetables and requires no cooking.

Blend together (use an electric blender or a sieve):
4 large, ripe tomatoes, peeled and chopped
1 medium cucumber, peeled and diced
1 medium onion, chopped
1 green pepper, seeded and chopped
1 cup tomato juice
1 tablespoon wine vinegar
3 tablespoons olive oil
1 small clove garlic
salt and pepper to taste

Chill well before serving. At serving time, pass bowls of:

chopped cucumber
chopped shallots
chopped green pepper
garlic croutons

These can be sprinkled on each portion of soup.

Chapter 14 • Meat

Meat has long been the staple element in our national diet and, although the fat content varies, meat is one of the main sources of fat in that diet. There are two types of fat in meat—separable and unseparable.

Separable fat, which is easily visible, can and must be cut away. To become efficient at this, keep a small, very sharp paring knife handy. A knife sharpener, used frequently, will keep the knife in prime condition and make this work easier. We also find that sitting down to trim the meat is less fatiguing and insures a more careful and complete job.

Unseparable fat is the thin, marbled layer of fat running through the bundles of meat fibers. Most people are unaware that this fat represents a tremendous source of fat intake. There is no way to trim this type of fat, yet it must be avoided as much as possible. It is for this reason that we emphasize the necessity for small meat servings or substitutions for meat at every opportunity.

Change Your Habits

It is most important to change your meat-eating habits. Meat must not be served more than three times each week and, even with this restriction, the portions should be kept to four to six ounces. Serving fish or poultry the rest of the week will provide adequate protein and control the amount of saturated fat you will eat.

Beef

Beef has the highest saturated fat content of all meats. Steaks and roasts that are heavily marbled should be served as infrequently as possible, and rib roasts and rib steaks are much too fatty to be used at all. If you want to serve steak occasionally, sirloin, tenderloin, and flank steak are the leanest. Carefully inspect the meat you buy to see which has the least amount of marbling. Luckily, the less expensive grade of beef is the healthiest. The most expensive grades of beef are often those that are most heavily marbled. These must be avoided if you are serious about helping your heart. Remember that heart disease caused by diet is a slow, relentless process that begins many years before a heart attack actually occurs.

Always use lean stewing beef when preparing stews, ragouts, or soups. Avoid short ribs (square flanken) because of their excess amounts of fat. Leaner types of meat often require more cooking to make them tender, but they are as nutritious as the fatty meats and are significantly better for you.

A good way to diminish meat intake is to "cheat" your family as the food industry does. You can do this by "padding" some meals. Many food processors add water, fat, or bread crumbs to meat, such as hamburger or canned meats. You can use this idea for better health and to improve the flavor of the meat. One way is to add a large amount of vegetables to stews. Another way is to add bread crumbs or vegetables to your meat when preparing a meat loaf. It is a good idea to use chopped lean veal mixed with beef when you make hamburgers, meat loaf, or meatballs since veal contains much less fat than beef. You won't alter the taste and your family will be eating less beef.

Never buy packaged hamburger meat, even though the price may be tempting, because you are probably getting a lot of waste fat. When you buy meat for hamburgers, buy only extra-lean ground beef. The best solution is to choose your own cut of lean beef and have the butcher trim and then grind the meat for you. We use round steak or lean stewing beef for this purpose. You may pay a little more, but it is your heart you are "treating."

When buying beef for oven or pot roasts, buy only the leanest cuts (those with the least marbling). Before you cook the roast, remove the cord, cut away all visible fat and then retie. Season as you normally would, then add a few tablespoons of oil to the pan so that the fat you have removed is replaced by a healthful fat.

Lamb

Lamb and mutton are in the same category as beef—high in saturated fat. If lamb is a favorite in your house, use only the leg or loin chops because they contain less fat than the other cuts. Again we must emphasize the importance of careful trimming *before* cooking. Any fat on the outside will soften and soak into the meat during cooking. Get rid of this unwanted fat before you cook so that it never gets to your table.

Pork

Some cuts of pork and ham are not as dangerous as lamb and beef because they contain less fat—this means less invisible fat. Only the leanest cuts of pork fillet and well-trimmed ham should be eaten;

even these should be eaten infrequently. Most other cuts of pork are very high in saturated fat. You can tell at a glance why you should never serve bacon! On infrequent occasions, Canadian or back bacon, very well trimmed, may be served. There are delicious bacon-tasting substitutes on the market. These come in a jar and can be used in place of crisp, crumbled bacon in such things as sandwiches, pizza, or dips.

Veal

Unlike beef, most cuts of veal have no marbling, so it is a simple job to just remove the separable fat. Veal is a low-fat meat with a minimum of waste. It can be prepared in such a variety of ways that it need never become monotonous. This section contains many recipes and you can easily adapt more from your own recipe book. Even the less expensive cuts of veal can be satisfactory. For stews, buy stewing veal and trim it yourself. When you want to use ground veal, do the same as you would for beef; choose the meat yourself and then have the butcher trim it well before grinding.

Organ and Variety Meats

Organ meats such as tongue, sweetbreads, kidney, or liver are high in cholesterol, so eat these sparingly, if at all. Never buy canned meats, sausages, hot dogs, or prepared meats for sandwiches, since you cannot control the fat content. Did you know that hot dogs may contain as much as 33 percent fat? When you look at a hot dog, think of it as two-thirds meat and one-third creamy, white fat.

Variety meats are great convenience foods, but it is a mistake to risk the health of your family to avoid a few minutes of work.

Cooking Hints

Defatting

Always cook a stew or ragout the day before using it so that you can chill the gravy. The fat will come to the top, and solidify; it is then easy to remove. Some natural gravies are delicious as is, but if you like yours thickened or seasoned just remember to remove the fat first.

Roasting and Broiling

When roasting or broiling, place your meat on a rack to allow the excess fat to drip off. This eliminates only some of the fat. When a steak is broiled and you see the fat drippings in the pan and you can no longer see the white, marbled fat in the meat, you may then assume that *all* the fat has broiled off. This is not true! Only the top part that is exposed to the heat has lost some of its fat—the rest is hidden inside the meat. You must remember that you are still eating a large amount of fat, even in a well-done steak.

Use a meat thermometer for oven roasting to insure that the meat is cooked to the right temperature. This will help prevent the meat from becoming too dry or overcooked, something that can easily happen when the fat is removed before cooking.

Browning

When a recipe calls for browning meat before adding other ingredients, try browning under the broiler instead of in a pan so that some of the fat will drip off. If you must brown in the pan, brown the well-trimmed meat in oil.

In the final analysis, meat, especially beef, represents a heavy source of our excess fat intake, and is a major cause of our diet problems. A great effort should be made to diminish overreliance on this type of food.

Remember:

1. Serve meat less often—increase your reliance on fish and poultry.
2. Trim your meat *before* cooking.
3. Serve smaller portions.

MEAT GUIDE SUMMARY

Most people enjoy meat as the basis of their main meal. However, meat is a major source of hard fat, and no matter how much you trim all visible fat, there still remains much fat in the form of marbling in some cuts of beef. This can be controlled by judicious selection of the meat you serve.

Choose and Trim Well	Avoid
Beef	*Beef*
Round steak	Rib steaks and roasts
Sirloin tip roast	Heavily marbled meat
Cube steak	Hot dogs
Rump or English roast	Preground hamburger meat
Flank steak	Tongue
Shank beef	Luncheon meats
Porterhouse steak	Short ribs
Tenderloin	
Lean stewing beef	

Choose and Trim Well	Avoid
Pork	*Pork*
Lean ham	Pigs feet
Canadian or back bacon	Bacon
Fillet of pork	Sausages
	Spareribs (use veal)
	Salt pork
Lamb	*Lamb*
Leg of lamb	Lamb shanks
Loin chops	Stewing lamb
	Breast
Veal	*Organ meats*
All veal	Brains
	Sweetbreads
	Liver
	Kidney

VEAL PATTIES

Combine:

2 pounds ground lean veal
¾ teaspoon salt
¼ teaspoon pepper
1 tablespoon Worcestershire sauce
1 egg
2 tablespoons water or broth
½ cup finely chopped onion

Shape into patties and pan fry or broil. At the last minute, add a little marinara or seasoned tomato sauce, if desired.

VEAL CHOPS AND SKILLET POTATOES

Trim all fat from: **6 rib or loin veal chops**

Dip them in: **1 egg (less ½ yolk)**

beaten with: **1 teaspoon water**

Then bread the
chops in: **¼ cup seasoned Italian bread crumbs**

(If plain crumbs are used, season them with salt, pepper, oregano, and garlic.)

Heat a skillet and fry chops uncovered over medium heat in:

¼ cup oil

about 20 minutes on each side.

Boil until tender in salted water, then set aside:

3 small potatoes, peeled and sliced

Remove the chops from the pan and mash potatoes in the oil and crumbs that remain in the pan, scraping the pan well. If the pan is too dry, add a few spoonfuls of the water the potatoes cooked in.

If you have to make more than your skillet can hold, brown the chops on each side quickly over high heat and place uncovered in a flat pan and bake in a 350° oven for 45 minutes.

BREADED VEAL SCALLOPS

Pound until thin:	**4 veal cutlets**
Sprinkle lightly with:	**salt and pepper to taste**
Dredge thoroughly with:	**flour**
Dip the floured cutlets in a mixture of:	**1 egg (less half the yolk)** **1 teaspoon water**
Coat the cutlets with:	**1 cup bread crumbs**

Refrigerate the breaded cutlets 1-2 hours to help the crumbs adhere to the meat while they are being cooked.

Heat in a large skillet:	**¼ cup oil**

Sauté the cutlets until golden brown on both sides. Arrange on a serving platter and serve immediately. Garnish with lemon wedges.

To add a little variation to this delicious meal, you can lay the cutlets on a platter, place a slice of lemon on each one, and top the lemon with a rolled fillet of anchovy. You could also arrange the cutlets on a bed of spaghetti and cover with a marinara sauce.

VEAL STEW BURGUNDY

Shake together in a paper bag:	**2 pounds well-trimmed veal pieces** **2 tablespoons flour** **½ teaspoon salt** **pepper**

Then brown the
floured veal in: **2 tablespoons oil**

Remove veal and set aside.

Add to the
remaining oil,
browning lightly: **1 small onion chopped very fine**
garlic to taste

Add: **⅔ cup chicken broth**
⅓ cup red wine
⅔ cup tomato juice
1 tablespoon chopped parsley
½ teaspoon rosemary

Cook slowly 10 minutes, and then return the meat. Continue cooking slowly, covered, for 1 hour or until tender. Serve with small whole or mashed potatoes.

VEAL STEW MARENGO

In a large skillet
heat: **4 tablespoons oil**

Brown: **3 pounds veal, well trimmed and cut into 2-inch**
cubes

Remove the veal with a slotted spoon and in the remaining oil brown:

2 large chopped onions

When onions are lightly browned, sprinkle in:

2 tablespoons flour

Cook the onions 3 or 4 minutes more.

Add: **1 15-ounce can stewed tomatoes**
1 teaspoon thyme
2 cloves crushed garlic
salt and pepper to taste

Put the veal in a casserole with the tomato mixture.

Then add: **1 cup dry white wine**
1 cup chicken broth (or enough broth to cover the
veal)
1 bay leaf
1 tablespoon chopped parsley

Bake covered in a 325° oven for 1 hour.

In a skillet sauté: **½ pound mushrooms**
1 can drained, tiny white onions

Add the mushrooms and onions to the stew and bake uncovered 45 minutes more. Garnish the stew with toast points.

VEAL SCALOPPINE WITH MUSHROOMS

Pound lightly until very thin:

1½-2 pounds of veal steaks

Dredge the veal with:

flour

Heat in a skillet: **¼ cup oil**

Add the veal and brown on both sides. Remove the veal from the pan.

Add: **½ pound fresh mushrooms, sliced**

and cook stirring for 2 or 3 minutes.

Combine: **2 cloves of minced garlic**
½ cup dry red wine
4 medium tomatoes, peeled and chopped
salt and freshly ground black pepper

Put the veal back into the skillet with the mushrooms and add the tomato-wine mixture. Simmer covered about 10 minutes (or until veal is tender). Garnish with parsley and serve immediately.

BAKED VEAL WITH EGGPLANT

Brown: **1½ pounds thinly sliced veal, well trimmed and**
lightly seasoned
1 large eggplant, cut in ¼-inch slices

in: **4 tablespoons oil**

In a lightly oiled baking dish, layer the veal and eggplant, alternating with:

8 ounces of marinara or meatless spaghetti sauce

Cover baking dish and bake in 350° oven for 45 minutes. Remove cover and bake 15 minutes longer. If desired, you can sprinkle some:

Italian flavored bread crumbs or
grated skim milk cheese

over the top for the last 15 minutes.

LAMB CURRY

Heat: **2 tablespoons oil**

Brown in oil and set aside:

2 pounds well-trimmed, cubed lamb

Sauté in the   **1 onion, chopped**
remaining oil: **2 stalks celery, chopped**
1 clove minced garlic

To this mixture add:	**1 10-ounce can mushroom gravy** **¼ cup water** **1 tablespoon tomato paste** **1 teaspoon curry powder** **salt and pepper to taste** **browned lamb**

Cover and simmer about one hour or until tender, and serve over hot rice. Pineapple rings are a delicious accompaniment to this dish.

LAMB KEBOBS

Trim carefully, and cut into two-inch cubes:

2 pounds lamb, well trimmed

Marinate for 2-3 hours in a mixture of:	**¼ cup oil** **1 teaspoon salt** **¼ teaspoon pepper** **2 tablespoons red wine**
Place the meat on skewers alternating with:	**small, whole mushrooms** **cherry tomatoes (or large, firm tomatoes cubed)** **cubes of green pepper** **raw or parboiled onions**

Broil until tender in your oven or on a barbecue. Keep kebobs about four inches from heat source, turning frequently.

EASTERN LAMB

Trim very well and cut into cubes:	**2 pounds lean lamb**
Combine the following and marinate the lamb for a few hours:	**1 teaspoon dry mustard** **1 teaspoon chili powder** **½ teaspoon ginger** **½ cup chopped onion** **½ teaspoon salt** **1 small clove garlic** **1 teaspoon turmeric** **¼ cup lemon juice** **1 teaspoon honey** **freshly ground black pepper**

The meat can be put on skewers or in a pan and broiled for about 15-20 minutes, turning occasionally. Serve over white rice with fruit such as canned pineapple slices or apricot halves.

PORK FILLET CHINESE STYLE

Cut on bias, into bite-sized pieces:

1 pound pork fillet

Marinate the meat for 15 minutes in:	**¼ teaspoon salt** **2 tablespoons soy sauce** **1 clove minced garlic** **¼ teaspoon ginger**
Heat in a large skillet:	**4 tablespoons oil**

Cook the meat covered for 5-8 minutes, stirring occasionally. Then slice thinly and add:

1 cup celery
1 cup green pepper
1 5-ounce can water chestnuts
2 large onions
½ pound fresh mushrooms

Combine and add:	**1 cup water** **2 tablespoons cornstarch** **2 teaspoons soy sauce**

Cook covered 5-10 minutes only; the vegetables will be crisp. If you wish, this may be prepared in advance up to the point of adding the cornstarch mixture.

SPAGHETTI MEAT SAUCE

This sauce takes a few extra minutes, but it is absolutely worth every minute. It freezes well, so make a large amount and have an instant supper on a busy day. This sauce is delicious on spaghetti, and is the base for lasagna.

Season:	**1 pound lean, minced beef** **1 pound lean, minced veal**
with:	**1 teaspoon salt** **¼ teaspoon pepper** **¼ teaspoon onion salt** **¼ teaspoon garlic salt** **1 tablespoon sugar** **½ teaspoon dry mustard** **2 tablespoons catsup**

Vary the amounts of seasoning to your own taste. Brown the meat in oil, then add the meat to the following sauce.

Sauce

Brown in oil:	**1 diced onion**
Add:	**1 48-ounce can tomato juice** **1 can tomato soup** **1 can tomato sauce**

1 can tomato paste
salt
pepper
2 tablespoons sugar
1 bay leaf
crushed chilies
½ teaspoon oregano
½ teaspoon paprika
1 clove minced garlic
¼ teaspoon basil

Simmer for 10 minutes, then add the seasoned meat and cook partially covered for several hours.

MEATLESS EGGPLANT SAUCE FOR SPAGHETTI

In a heavy saucepan sauté until golden:
¼ cup oil
½ cup finely chopped onion
1 clove garlic, crushed

Add and continue cooking and stirring for 5 minutes:
1 medium eggplant cut into half-inch cubes (about 3 cups)
1 small green pepper, slivered

Then add:
3 cups peeled, chopped tomatoes
¼ teaspoon dried basil
½ teaspoon mixed Italian spice
½ teaspoon salt
pepper

Cover and simmer 30 minutes.

Then add:
½ cup slivered ripe olives
6 anchovies chopped very finely
1 tablespoon capers, chopped

Continue cooking 5 minutes longer. Taste and add more salt if necessary.

Toss:
hot spaghetti

with:
1 tablespoon oil
1 tablespoon chopped parsley

Pour onto deep platter and pour eggplant sauce over.

Sprinkle lightly with:
grated skim milk cheese

MEAT LOAF

Combine:
1 pound lean ground veal
1 pound lean ground beef
1 can of vegetarian vegetable soup

½ cup bread crumbs
½ cup chopped onion
1 tablespoon Worcestershire sauce
1 egg, slightly beaten
1 teaspoon salt
¼ teaspoon pepper

You can also add any other cooked vegetable—maybe leftovers from last night's dinner.

Place the meat in a loaf pan or in a loaf shape in a roasting pan. Bake in 350° oven for about one hour. Spread catsup over top last 15 minutes of cooking. For a small family, divide into 3 loaves, cook one, freeze two—allow longer baking time if you were not able to thaw before baking.

MEAT LASAGNA

Arrange in layers in a lightly oiled 7 x 11 inch baking dish, starting with a thin layer of sauce:

2 cups meat sauce
⅓ pound lasagna noodles (boiled in salted water and drained)
½ pound cottage cheese
4 ounces skim milk mozzarella cheese grated or broken in bits

Repeat the layers twice. The final layer of cheese is covered with one more layer of noodles and a thin covering of sauce. Bake for 30 minutes in a 350° oven. Let stand for 5 minutes to settle. Cut and serve.

This lasagna can be prepared ahead and frozen. Allow to come to room temperature before baking.

These are the measurements for our favorite baking dish. You can vary the amounts of the ingredients to suit your individual taste.

MOUSAKA (GREEK CASSEROLE)

Sauté until golden:	1 medium onion, chopped fine, in 2 tablespoons oil
Add and brown:	1 pound lean ground beef
Add and simmer 5 minutes:	1 6-ounce can tomato paste ¾ cup water
Add the following and simmer gently until sauce is thickened, (½ hour):	2 teaspoons salt ⅛ teaspoon pepper pinch cinnamon pinch nutmeg pinch cloves

⅛ teaspoon thyme
1 teaspoon oregano
½ cup dry red wine
½ cup mushrooms cooked or canned (optional)

Slice ½ inch thick, but do not peel:
1 medium-sized eggplant
or
4 medium-sized potatoes, peeled

(If potatoes are used, cover with cold water and bring to a boil, drain.) Layer meat mixture and eggplant (or potatoes) in lightly oiled casserole, ending with the vegetable. Sprinkle each layer of vegetables with salt.

In a small saucepan make a mixture of:
2 tablespoons flour
1 cup skim milk
¼ teaspoon salt
2 tablespoons oil
⅛ teaspoon pepper

Cook over low heat, stirring constantly until thickened.

In a small bowl beat:

1 egg, less half yolk

Add about half the hot sauce to the egg, stirring constantly, then return the egg and sauce mixture to saucepan. Continue cooking, stirring constantly for one minute longer. Pour over meat and vegetables in casserole and bake uncovered 45-60 minutes in 350° oven, or until brown and bubbly. Serve from casserole.

STUFFED GREEN PEPPERS

Cut in half lengthwise, remove core and seeds from:

4 firm green peppers

and set aside.

Sauté until golden:
3 tablespoons chopped onion in
2 tablespoons oil

Remove from heat and add:
½ pound lean ground beef
½ cup "5-minute rice" (raw)
½ cup tomato juice or water
½ teaspoon salt

Fill pepper cases with meat mixture and place in shallow baking dish.

Pour:
1½ cups marinara or meatless spaghetti sauce

over the stuffed peppers. Bake covered in 350° oven for 45 minutes, then uncovered for another 15 minutes. To brown, baste tops often after uncovering. Any additional meat may be rolled into balls and dropped into the tomato sauce.

SKILLET ZUCCHINI AND BEEF

In a large skillet over medium heat sauté until tender:
- 1 medium onion, finely chopped
- 1 green pepper, finely chopped
- 1 tablespoon oil

Add:
- 1 pound lean ground beef

Keep stirring until meat is brown.

Stir in:
- 1 16-ounce can stewed tomatoes
- 1 6-ounce can tomato paste
- 1 teaspoon salt
- ½ teaspoon oregano
- ¼ teaspoon garlic powder

Simmer covered 10 minutes.

Add:
- 2 medium zucchini cut into ¼-inch slices

Continue cooking covered another 10-15 minutes until zucchini is tender-crisp. This serves four.

SALISBURY STEAK WITH ONION SAUCE

Heat:
- 2 tablespoons oil

Add:
- 5 medium onions, peeled and sliced

Cook onions 2 minutes stirring occasionally.

Mix and add:
- 1½ cups cold water
- 3 tablespoons soy sauce
- ½ teaspoon sugar

Bring to a boil and then cook over medium heat 10 minutes until onions are tender.

Dissolve:
- 1 tablespoon cornstarch

in:
- ¼ cup water

and slowly stir the cornstarch mixture into onions until sauce thickens. Set aside and keep warm.

Season:
- 1½ pounds lean ground beef

Shape into patties and broil as desired. Put patties on a platter and spoon the cooked onions over them. Serve hot.

PEPPER STEAK

Slice very thin, across the grain:
- 1 flank steak

Combine and pour over the meat:
- 5 tablespoons soy sauce
- 2 tablespoons sherry

                        1 tablespoon sugar
                        1 tablespoon cornstarch

Set aside for 30 minutes.

Then heat: **2 tablespoons oil**

Add: **1 green pepper, sliced**
                        6 scallions cut in slices lengthwise
                        3 tomatoes, quartered

Cook the vegetables for 2 or 3 minutes only, so that they do not lose their crispness. Remove the vegetables from the pan.

To the pan add: **½ teaspoon ginger**
                        the marinated meat

Cook until the meat is brown, about 5 minutes, stirring often. Add the cooked vegetables until they are heated through. Serve over hot white rice.

BROILED FLANK STEAK

Marinate for several hours or overnight:

                        1 well-trimmed flank steak

in a mixture of: **4 tablespoons soy sauce**
                        2 tablespoons water
                        1 small onion, chopped
                        1 tablespoon parsley (fresh if possible)

Broil to desired degree of doneness. Slice thinly on an angle across the grain and serve at once.

TERIYAKI STEAK

Marinate 6 hours: **1 well-trimmed flank steak**

in a mixture of: **¼ cup soy sauce**
                        1 teaspoon brown sugar
                        1 tablespoon Worcestershire sauce
                        1 teaspoon vinegar
                        ¾ teaspoon ginger

Pierce steak with fork and turn once or twice during marinating time. Broil as desired. Remove steak and pour remaining marinade in pan to heat. Slice steak across grain—place on heated platter and pour hot marinade over. Serve with rice.

SUKIYAKI FROM LEFTOVERS

Mix thoroughly: **2 teaspoons cornstarch**
                        ¾ cup water

Add and set aside: **2 tablespoons soy sauce**
¼ cup catsup

In: **2 tablespoons oil**

Sauté until
translucent: **1 large onion, chopped**

Add: **2 stalks celery, sliced on the diagonal**
½ green pepper sliced

Add the soy mixture and cook over medium heat for about 5 minutes, stirring constantly. Just before serving, add leftover:

broiled flank steak, sliced very thin

The flank steak should not be recooked, only heated through. Serve over a bed of white rice.

This is such a favorite in our family that we serve flank steak in order to have leftovers for the sukiyaki.

SPICY POT ROAST
(PAN BARBECUED STEAK)

Combine and
set aside: **1 can tomato soup**
2 tablespoons brown sugar
2 teaspoons prepared mustard
2 tablespoons Worcestershire sauce
2 teaspoons lemon juice
½ teaspoon salt
¼ teaspoon pepper

In a heavy pot, **3-4 pound boneless pot roast of beef (top,**
sear on all sides: **bottom, or eye round) very well trimmed**

Be sure meat is evenly browned. Remove meat from pot and remove any fat that has collected. Return meat to the pot and cover with:

tomato soup mixture

Partially cover pot and simmer slowly for 2-3 hours or until tender. Turn the meat a few times during cooking. Refrigerate overnight with the gravy separate. When ready to serve, skim fat from gravy (if there is any), slice meat, return to the gravy, and heat through. Serve with mashed potatoes and a delectable vegetable.

BEEF STEW

Trim very carefully: **2 pounds stewing beef**

Shake beef in a paper bag with:

2 tablespoons flour

In a heavy pot sauté until golden:	**3 tablespoons oil** **2 small onions, cut fine**
Add:	**floured beef** **salt and pepper to taste** **¼ teaspoon paprika** **¼ bunch fresh dill or 1 tablespoon dried dill weed (optional)**

Cook covered slowly as water evaporates. Allow meat to *nearly* burn. Stir often. Then add water to make a delicious, rich, brown gravy. If desired, parboiled celery, carrots, and potatoes may be added to finish cooking in the gravy.

GOLFER'S STEW

Arrange in layers in casserole:	**2 pounds lean stewing meat** **2 potatoes, peeled and cut into chunks** **2 stalks of celery cut into 2-inch pieces** **4 carrots peeled and cut into 1-inch pieces** **1 bay leaf** **1 can of tomato soup or canned tomatoes** **2 tablespoons water** **salt and pepper to taste**

Seal with two layers of aluminum foil and place cover over foil, taking care not to tear foil. Bake in 250° oven for 7 hours. Before serving add 1 can of small peas. This is a marvelous meal for that day out of the kitchen.

BEEF STROGANOFF

Trim and cut into slices ½ inch thick:	
	1½ pounds beef fillet
Season with:	**salt and pepper**
Heat:	**2 tablespoons oil**

Add the meat and brown quickly on both sides. Remove the meat to a platter and keep hot.

In a saucepan, heat:	**2 tablespoons oil**
Add, stirring until well blended:	
	1 tablespoon flour
Add:	**1 cup very hot beef broth or consommé**

Add the broth all at once to the oil-flour mixture, stirring vigorously until the sauce is thick and smooth.

Stir in:	**1 teaspoon prepared mustard**

Add: **3 tablespoons "sour cream" (see recipe) or natural-flavored skim milk yogurt**

Heat slowly for 3 minutes. Do not allow the sauce to boil since it will curdle. Pour over the meat and serve at once.

OVEN ROASTS

Do not buy meat that is heavily marbled with fat. Untie the roast, remove all visible fat and retie. Using about 2 tablespoons per pound of meat:

oil

the roast, and then sprinkle liberally with a mixture of:

2 tablespoons flour
1 tablespoon salt
½ teaspoon pepper
4 teaspoons paprika
1 teaspoon garlic powder
½ teaspoon dry mustard

(Store remaining mixture in a covered spice jar for future use.)

Roast the meat according to taste. Half an hour before serving, remove meat, retain the drippings, but pour off all fat that comes to the top of the drippings.

Return the meat to the pan and place under it:

1 small onion, very finely chopped

Return to the oven for about 20 minutes or until the onions brown slightly. Add to the pan:

½ cup water

and blend vigorously, scraping with rubber scraper until all the drippings are dissolved.

Taste and add more seasonings if necessary. Return to the oven until serving time.

GENERAL INSTRUCTIONS FOR OVEN ROASTS AND GRAVIES

Do not use rib roasts or any cuts or legs that are too heavily marbled with fat. Untie meat, remove all visible fat and retie.

Rub meat with: **oil**
                      season as usual

Place in pan and cover meat with a double layer of cheesecloth.

Over this pour: **oil (about 1 teaspoon per pound of meat)**

Roast in your usual way. Make gravy as you usually do, using defatted drippings.

SAUTÉED CHICKEN LIVERS

Sauté until golden: **2 tablespoons oil**
2 large onions cut in half and then sliced ¼ inch thick
1 green pepper, sliced (optional)
salt, pepper, paprika to taste

Add: **1 pound chicken livers (well washed and trimmed carefully of any green veins that have been left, since they will give your livers a bitter taste)**

Cover and continue cooking 10-15 minutes, stirring often until livers are no longer pink inside. Do not overcook because this toughens them.

½ pound sautéed mushrooms may be added

Serve in toast baskets or on rice.

BORDELAISE SAUCE FOR TENDERLOIN STEAK

Heat: **2 tablespoons oil**
Add: **2 tablespoons flour**

mixing well until flour is brown.

Gradually stir in: **2 cups beef or chicken stock**
2 cloves garlic, minced
2 tablespoons chopped onions
1 bay leaf
1 tablespoon catsup
1 tablespoon Worcestershire sauce
½ teaspoon celery salt

Simmer for 5 minutes. Strain and then add:

3 tablespoons cooking sherry

Serve hot.

RED WINE AND MUSHROOM SAUCE

In: **2 tablespoons oil**
Sauté until golden: **2 thinly sliced onions**
½ pound thinly sliced mushrooms
Add: **1½ cups beef bouillon**
½ cup dry red wine

Simmer for 15 minutes.

Stir a little of the wine mixture into:

2 tablespoons flour

Then return this to the wine mixture. Return to a boil stirring constantly. Add salt to taste. Serve hot over broiled steak.

Chapter 15 • Poultry

Thank goodness for poultry! It is versatile, nutritious, relatively inexpensive, and makes an excellent substitute for beef. Acceptable poultry includes chicken, turkey, squab, and Cornish hen. Duck and goose must be avoided because they contain too much fat.

No matter how you prepare poultry, all visible fat must be removed *before* cooking. If it is left on to be removed later, the fat will soak into the meat during the cooking process and then can never be removed. The fat under the skin appears as easily visible pads. Once these are removed, the remaining skin may be eaten.

The breast or white meat contains no saturated fat. The dark meat does contain some, but it is still much healthier than beef. Supermarkets today sell sectioned poultry, which makes it easier to serve each member of the family his favorite portion.

Chicken, especially the breast, is ideally suited for a low-fat diet. There is no limit to the ways you can prepare it; you must have many favorite recipes that can be used on our program. Most of these can easily be adapted for healthful eating. Just remember to brown in oil rather than butter, remove all visible fat, and avoid sauces made with cream. Substitute yogurt or skim milk to make a "cream" sauce that you may eat safely.

Hints on Preparation

For convenience, it is a good idea to cook chicken breasts in advance. They can be deboned and frozen in small portions and will then be ready for use in such things as chicken sandwiches, salads, or "creamed" chicken.

When buying turkey, never buy one that is deep basted or prebasted. The latter type has been injected with coconut oil, lard, or butter, all of which are saturated fats. Our mothers made delicious turkey without prebasting and so can we. To make a nicely browned turkey, rub it with a mixture of 1 tablespoon paprika and ½ cup oil. Remember that white turkey meat is practically fat free and much less fattening than most cuts of beef or lamb. Buy a large bird and you will have leftovers for low-fat lunches and dinners—especially if you make use of your freezer.

Check your favorite stuffing recipe. Substitute for any undesirable ingredients; for instance, use oil instead of melted butter or lard. Try our delicious recipes for healthful stuffings if you don't have your own.

Giblets must not be eaten because they are organ meats very high in cholesterol. They may be used only for preparing stock or broth, but remember to discard the giblets after cooking, chill the broth, and remove any fat that comes to the top.

Most wild game is low in saturated fat—this includes pheasant, quail, rabbit, and venison. No doubt these are not regular fare for most of us, but they make a nice change for a special dinner.

ROASTED CHICKEN

This method may be used for small broilers or chicken parts.

Place lean, well-trimmed chicken on a flat pan. Do not crowd the chicken. Brush the skin with:

oil

Season with:
salt
pepper
paprika
garlic salt or powder

Place:
1 medium onion, chopped

under the chicken. Place the chicken in a 400° oven uncovered and roast for 1 hour or more if whole chickens are used. The last half hour, baste very frequently, adding a little water if needed. This method is the one we use in all recipes requiring precooked chicken. Remove any fat from the gravy that is left and freeze it until needed. It makes a marvelous base for stews, meatballs, and so on.

JAVANESE CHICKEN

Split and remove all visible fat from:
4-6 chicken breasts

Dredge the chicken with:
¼ cup flour, seasoned with salt and pepper

In heavy frying pan heat:
4 tablespoons oil

Brown chicken gently and place in a casserole.

To the remaining oil add:
1 clove garlic, crushed
2 medium onions, chopped
½ pound mushrooms, sliced

Sauté until tender, but not brown.

Add:
          2 cups canned Italian tomatoes
          2 green peppers chopped
          ½ teaspoon salt
          ¼ teaspoon curry powder
          ¼ teaspoon thyme
          ¼ teaspoon cayenne pepper
          ½ cup dried currants or raisins

Simmer for 5 minutes. Pour over chicken, cover, and bake for one hour in a 325° oven. Serve on a bed of white rice, garnished with toasted, slivered almonds.

OVEN-FRIED CHICKEN

Remove all fat
from: **2 small chickens cut up or 4 chicken breasts**

Dip the chicken in: **½ cup oil**

covering all sides. Then roll the chicken pieces in a mixture of:

          1 cup dried bread crumbs
          2 teaspoons salt
          ¼ teaspoon pepper

Place chicken in a shallow pan and bake in a 350° oven for about one hour, or until the chicken is tender and brown. This chicken can be served either hot or cold and it is delicious for a picnic lunch.

STIR-FRY CHICKEN

Skin and debone: **2 whole chicken breasts**

Cut each one across the grain into ¼-inch strips.

Heat: **2 tablespoons oil**

Add chicken strips and cook while stirring until they turn white. This takes about three minutes.

To the chicken add: **1 green pepper cut into strips**
          1 small onion, halved and then sliced ¼-inch thick
          1 cup of celery strips
          1 5-ounce can of water chestnuts, drained
            and thinly sliced
          ½ cup chicken broth
          1 teaspoon salt
          ¼ teaspoon ginger

Cover and cook 7 minutes.

Mix until smooth: **1 tablespoon cornstarch**
2 tablespoons soy sauce
¼ cup water

Add to skillet. Turn down heat to low. Simmer uncovered for about three minutes, stirring occasionally. Serve over a bed of rice.

STUFFED HALF BROILER

Place on flat pan, skin side up: **4 small broiler halves or large quarters (well trimmed)**

Brush with: **oil**

Season with: **salt**
pepper
paprika

Place about two inches from broiler and broil until brown, basting frequently. Meanwhile prepare half a recipe of Bread Stuffing. Turn chicken and spoon stuffing over bone side. Brush with oil. Bake in 400° oven uncovered (stuffing side up) for about 1 hour. Baste exposed chicken skin frequently, add a little water if necessary.

ORIENTAL CHICKEN KEBOBS

Skin, debone, and cut each into 16 pieces:

2 whole chicken breasts

Marinate the chicken in a mixture of the following for 1 hour:

1 tablespoon yogurt
¼ teaspoon salt
¼ teaspoon turmeric
⅛ teaspoon dry mustard
½ teaspoon curry powder
1 teaspoon lemon juice
1 teaspoon vinegar

Then thread on 4 skewers, alternating chicken pieces with:

8 small onions
8 small tomatoes

Broil slowly over hot coals or in a kitchen broiler for about 10 minutes or until the chicken is cooked. Place on a platter, sprinkle with lemon juice and garnish with green pepper rings and fresh parsley.

CHICKEN WITH BING CHERRY SAUCE

Season: **4 chicken breasts (well trimmed)**
salt and pepper

Place the chicken in a shallow roasting pan skin side up and brush it with:

2 tablespoons oil

Broil the chicken until brown. Combine the following ingredients thoroughly:

1 cup water
½ cup raisins
½ cup brown sugar
1 teaspoon garlic salt
2 medium onions, sliced thinly
1 11-ounce bottle chili sauce
1 tablespoon Worcestershire sauce

Pour these ingredients over the chicken and cover the whole pan with aluminum foil. Bake for 1½ hours in a 350° oven. Remove the foil and add:

1 14-ounce can bing cherries, drained
1 cup sherry

Roast for an additional 15 minutes basting frequently. Place the chicken on a platter and pour the sauce over it.

FOIL-BAKED CHICKEN

With no broiler pan to clean up this chicken is doubly good.

Cut into portions and spread in a large, flat, foil-lined pan:

3-4 pounds of chicken pieces (we suggest breasts only)

Combine and pour over chicken:

2 teaspoons dry mustard
2 teaspoons chili powder
2 teaspoons paprika
2 teaspoons salt
2 tablespoons lemon juice
2 tablespoons Worcestershire sauce
4 tablespoons oil
¼ cup brown sugar
⅓ cup vinegar
⅓ cup catsup
½ cup water

Cover chicken with another piece of foil. Bake in a 400° oven for 45 minutes. Remove foil cover, and bake 15-20 minutes longer, basting often. Place the chicken on a platter, spoon remaining sauce over it, and serve at once.

CHINESE CHICKEN

Place:

1 chicken, well trimmed, cut into serving pieces, and lightly salted

skin side up in a large baking dish.

Combine the following and pour over the chicken:	**2 teaspoons cornstarch mixed with** **⅓ cup water** **⅓ cup vinegar** **¼ teaspoon salt** **⅓ cup sugar** **½ teaspoon monosodium glutamate** **1 tablespoon oil** **1 tablespoon catsup** **1 small can pineapple cubes**

Bake uncovered in 350° oven for 1 hour.

Then add:	**1 green pepper cut into strips**

Continue baking for ½-¾ hour longer, basting frequently. Add more water if sauce becomes too thick. Fifteen minutes before serving add:

2 tomatoes cut in wedges

Serve over white rice. This chicken is as good as many a Chinese restaurant will serve.

CHICKEN WITH ARTICHOKE HEARTS

Place in paper bag:	**2 tablespoons flour** **½ teaspoon salt** **⅛ teaspoon pepper**

Add, and shake until chicken is evenly covered:

3 whole chicken breasts, split and all fat removed

Brown in:	**¼ cup oil**
Reduce heat and add:	**¾ cup sherry** **¾ cup chicken broth**

Cover and cook for 45 minutes.

Add:	**1 package frozen artichoke hearts** **2 tomatoes cut in wedges** **1 medium onion, sliced thinly** **1 medium green pepper, sliced**
Sprinkle with:	**salt to taste**

Cover and cook 15 minutes longer.

ALMOND-ORANGE CHICKEN

In a large skillet heat:	**2 tablespoons oil**
Brown well on all sides:	**3 whole chicken breasts, halved, with all fat removed**

Stir in:
1½ cups orange juice
1 teaspoon poultry seasoning (optional)
1½ teaspoons salt

Reduce heat, cover, and simmer for 30 minutes or until chicken is fork tender, basting occasionally with the liquid in the skillet. Remove the chicken to a heated platter and keep warm.

Combine:
2 tablespoons cornstarch
2 tablespoons water

Gradually stir this mixture into the hot liquid in the skillet. Cook, stirring constantly, until sauce is thickened and clear.

Stir in:
½ cup slivered almonds
or
½ cup chopped walnuts

Pour sauce over the chicken and serve immediately.

CASSEROLE CHICKEN

This is one of those delicious one-dish meals.

Shake together in a paper bag:
½ cup flour
½ teaspoon salt
¼ teaspoon pepper
3 pounds of chicken pieces, well trimmed

Remove the chicken pieces and brown them in:

¼ cup oil

Place the chicken in a casserole.

In the remaining oil, sauté:
1 medium onion, finely cut
¼ cup green pepper, thinly sliced
½ cup celery, sliced diagonally

Add and heat through:
1½ cups whole tomatoes (canned or fresh)
1 teaspoon chicken soup mix
¾ cup carrots sliced diagonally

Pour this mixture over the chicken. Bake covered about 1 hour in 350° oven. Add a little tomato juice if necessary. Ten minutes before serving add:

1 small can mushrooms
1 small can whole, cooked potatoes

LEMON-MUSTARD CHICKEN

Make a mixture of:
¼ cup lemon juice
2 teaspoons oil
2 teaspoons prepared mustard

Brush both sides of:
4 chicken breasts (well trimmed)

with this mixture and marinate for 2 hours. Preheat broiler to very hot and broil bone side up, close to the heat for 5 minutes. Place on lower rack and broil for 5 minutes more. Turn the chicken pieces and repeat the process. The complete cooking process should take about 20 minutes and the chicken should be charred on the outside and juicy inside.

CHICKEN MARENGO

Combine in a
paper bag and
shake well:

½ cup flour
1 teaspoon salt
½ teaspoon freshly ground black pepper
1 teaspoon dried tarragon
3 pounds chicken, well trimmed and cut into serving
    pieces

Reserve the remaining flour.

Heat in a large skillet:

½ cup oil

Brown chicken pieces on all sides. Remove the chicken and place in a heavy casserole.

Add: 1½ tablespoons of the reserved flour

to the oil remaining in the skillet. Gradually stir in:

1 cup dry white wine

Stirring constantly, continue cooking until the sauce is thickened and smooth. Pour the sauce over the chicken and add:

2 cups canned tomatoes
1 clove garlic finely chopped
½ pound mushrooms sliced

Cover the casserole and bake in a 350° oven until the chicken is tender, about 1 hour.

Sprinkle with: chopped parsley

Serve hot and garnish with small, peeled apricot halves sitting on small pineapple slices.

SWEET AND PUNGENT CHICKEN

Mix together in saucepan and bring to a boil for one minute:

½ cup pineapple juice
¼ cup juice of sweet mixed pickles
2 tablespoons soy sauce
shake of garlic powder

Add: 6 pieces of the sweet mixed pickles, sliced thin
6 slices of pineapple, cut up

2 cooked breasts of chicken, cut up in pieces
2 teaspoons cornstarch dissolved in
2 tablespoons water

Cook slowly until thick, stirring constantly.

Add: 1 tomato, cut in wedges

Continue cooking until tomato is heated through. Serve at once over a bed of rice.

CHICKEN WITH ALMONDS

In a skillet heat: ¼ cup oil

Add, browning on all sides:

3-4 chicken breasts, well trimmed

Remove the chicken and keep hot. To the pan add:

1 clove garlic chopped
2 tablespoons chopped onion

Cook gently for 3 minutes. Add the following and stir until mixture is smooth:

1 tablespoon tomato paste
2 tablespoons flour

Then add: 1½ cups chicken broth
2 tablespoons sherry

When the mixture comes to a boil, return the chicken to the pan and add:

2 tablespoons slivered almonds
1 teaspoon dried tarragon
salt and pepper to taste

Cover and simmer slowly for 45-60 minutes, adding a little water if necessary. Transfer the chicken to a shallow casserole.

Stir: ¾ cup "sour cream" (see recipe) or natural-flavored skim milk yogurt

into the sauce remaining in the pan and heat thoroughly, being careful not to boil. Pour the sauce over the chicken and brown lightly under the broiler.

SWEET AND PUNGENT CHICKEN AND MEATBALLS

To: ½ pound very lean ground beef

Add: 1 slice white bread (with crusts cut off) that has been completely soaked in water and not drained
1 large carrot, finely grated
salt and pepper to taste

Lightly roll into balls and set aside.

In a heavy pot heat:	2 tablespoons oil
Add and sauté:	1 medium onion, cut fine
Add:	1 can tomato soup or sauce
	2 tablespoons brown sugar
	2 tablespoons lemon juice
	¼ cup seedless raisins

Add the meatballs and:

2 breasts of chicken, deboned, skinned, and cut into pieces

Simmer partially covered 1-1½ hours.

CHICKEN À LA KING

Prepare:	2 cups basic cream sauce (see chapter 12)
Add:	1 cup chicken stock

Stir until smooth and keep hot.

Sauté:	1 green pepper, sliced
	1 cup mushrooms, sliced
	2 tablespoons oil

Add to the sauce.

Then stir in:	¼ cup sherry (optional)
Season with:	salt
	pepper
	paprika
Add:	2 cups chicken pieces, diced
	4 tablespoons pimento, chopped

Serve over rice, toast points, or in toast baskets.

Garnish with:	chopped parsley

CHICKEN LASAGNA

This makes a large lasagna and is perfect for a big party.

Remove skin, debone, and cut into bite-size pieces:

1 small, cooked chicken

Prepare:	2 cups cream sauce (see recipe)
	2 packages frozen, chopped spinach, cooked as directed on package and drained
	1 large jar meatless marinara or spaghetti sauce (30 ounces)
	1 package lasagna noodles, cooked
	½ pound cottage cheese

In a 9 x 12 inch baking dish make layers of:

marinara sauce
lasagna noodles
marinara sauce
cream sauce
cottage cheese
chopped spinach
chicken

Repeat once more, ending with a layer of lasagna noodles. Bake, covered with foil, in 350° oven for ½ hour.

Top with: **shredded skim milk mozzarella cheese**

Continue baking another ½ hour uncovered. This may be prepared in 2 or more smaller pans and frozen unbaked. Thaw before baking.

PAELLA

This is a very good buffet dish since it can be made in a large quantity—but remember that any left over will freeze beautifully.

Prepare and set aside:
3 pounds raw chicken, cut into serving pieces and seasoned with salt and pepper
1½-2 pounds shrimp, shelled, cleaned, and deveined (scallops, lobster meat, or shrimp-sized pieces of fillet may be used instead of or in addition to the shrimp)

In a heavy skillet heat:

⅓ cup oil

Add: **the pieces of chicken**

and cook over moderate heat until brown and partially cooked (10-15 minutes). Remove from pan.

Then add:
1 cup chopped onion
1 clove minced garlic

Cook about 10 minutes over low heat or until the onion is transparent.

Bring to a boil in a large saucepan:

4 cups chicken broth

and then add: **the cleaned shrimp or other seafood**

Cook covered for 3 minutes, and uncovered for 3 minutes longer.

To the broth mixture, add:
½ teaspoon white pepper
3 teaspoons salt

½ teaspoon thyme
½ teaspoon paprika
½ teaspoon oregano
1 teaspoon saffron

        2 cups canned tomatoes
        ½ pound sliced mushrooms
        browned chicken pieces

If you want to prepare the paella in advance, set it aside at this point and refrigerate the mixture until needed.

When you are ready to finish the dish, add to the chicken mixture:

        2 cups raw rice (not the quick-cooking type)
        1 package defrosted frozen or fresh peas
        1 can artichoke hearts

Mix thoroughly and place in a lightly oiled 4- or 5-quart casserole or paella dish. Bake covered in 375° oven for 1¼ hours or until all the liquid has been absorbed. Stir once or twice during the cooking.

Garnish with: **12 steamed clams (optional)**
                    strips of pimento
                    sliced, stuffed olives

This serves 8-10.

BREAD STUFFING

Sauté until golden: **1 medium opion, chopped finely, in**
                        2 tablespoons oil

Add: **2 stalks and leaves of celery, cut finely**

Season with: **½ teaspoon salt**
                        pepper to taste

Remove crusts and soak in water until soft:

        1 small loaf of day-old bread (12 ounces)

Squeeze out gently and place in large bowl with onion mixture.

Add: **2 egg whites**
                    1 egg yolk

and beat until smooth. Fill cavity of turkey or chicken loosely.

SWEET POTATO STUFFING

Sauté until golden: **2 medium onions, chopped finely, in**
                        2 tablespoons oil

Add: **1 pound sweet potatoes, mashed**
                    2 cups crushed Grape Nut Flakes
                    2 beaten eggs
                    salt and pepper to taste
                    a little hot water

Stuff turkey cavity loosely. Any extra stuffing can be put in aluminum foil and baked for one hour.

Chapter 16 • Fish

Fish is a particularly desirable food for our purposes. It is high in protein, low in saturated fat, and, as an added bonus, it has half the calories of an equal amount of the leanest meat. Therefore, fish should be eaten several times a week for lunch or dinner.

There is such a large variety of fish available today, thanks to the speed of delivery and to the increased use of the freezer, that it is easy to plan many menus based on this very healthful food.

The reason some people show a lack of interest in fish is that it is often not properly prepared, rather, it is usually overcooked. Fish is naturally tender and requires very little cooking. Once you can tell exactly when the fish is done, all your fish dishes should be successful. When properly cooked, the shiny look will disappear and the flesh will look white and opaque. It should be moist and flake easily with a fork. To achieve this, prepare your fish only at the last minute—never cook it in advance and reheat it, this will make it dry.

Be extra careful when selecting commercially frozen fish preparations. Many are predipped in batter or crumbs in which lard or shortening has been used. Remember to check the labels for this. Don't get caught in the trap of eating unsuspected fats just when you think you are doing the opposite with a fish meal. When in doubt, it is always better and cheaper to prepare your own.

There are many ways to prepare fish, most of which are simple and require little time. If you are in the habit of dotting fish with butter, try sprinkling it with a little oil instead. You will obtain the taste you like, but will avoid the dangers of butter.

There is still a great deal of controversy over the status of shellfish in this type of diet. Although they have a low saturated fat content, they are high in cholesterol. We feel that they can be eaten, but only on occasion. Caviar and roe are also in this category.

Canned fish is convenient to use and is readily available in many varieties. This makes a fast, easy, protein-rich meal for lunch or dinner and is especially useful when you are short of time.

We have taken extra care to provide a comprehensive range of fish recipes in this book. Use this food generously and treat your heart to good meals.

OVEN-BAKED FISH

Season:	**2 pounds fish fillets (sole, perch, or haddock)**
With:	**salt and pepper**
Dip the fish in:	**oil**
and coat with:	**1 cup bread crumbs or corn flake crumbs**

Place fish on a lightly oiled baking dish in a single layer. Bake in a 350° oven for 30 minutes or until fish flakes easily. Serve with tartar sauce and lemon wedges.

OVEN-FRIED FILLETS

Combine:	**¼ cup dry bread crumbs**
	¼ teaspoon salt
	dash of pepper
	⅛ teaspoon thyme
	⅛ teaspoon oregano
Brush both sides of:	**1 pound of fish fillets, fresh or frozen**
with:	**2 tablespoons of prepared mustard**

Then dip in crumbs, and place on lightly oiled baking sheet.

Sprinkle with:	**2 tablespoons oil**

Bake in 500° oven 10 minutes, or until cooked.

FILLET BAKED IN "CREAM" OF MUSHROOM SOUP

Place in a lightly oiled baking dish and set aside:

	1 pound fillets, lightly salted
Prepare:	**1 cup white sauce (see chapter 12)**

Sauté in oil and add to the white sauce:

	½ cup mushrooms
	1 clove minced garlic (optional)

Pour the sauce over the fish. Place in a 350° oven and bake 15 minutes or until the fish flakes easily. Serve at once.

HAWAIIAN FISH

Dip:	**1 pound fish fillets**
in:	**skim milk**
and then dust fish with:	
	flour

Sauté fish in: **1 tablespoon oil**

Set aside and keep hot.

Sauté: **2 tablespoons oil**
1 stalk celery, finely sliced
¼ green pepper, finely sliced
2 scallions, finely cut

Combine the following and add to the vegetable mixture:

5 tablespoons brown sugar
1 small can pineapple tidbits and juice
1 teaspoon cornstarch (dissolved in pineapple juice)
¼ teaspoon ginger
3 tablespoons catsup

Simmer until slightly thickened and clear. Place the fish on a bed of rice and pour the sauce over it.

SWEET AND PUNGENT BAKED FISH WITH PINEAPPLE

Sauté for 5 minutes until golden: **2 tablespoons oil**
1 green pepper, cut in strips
1 medium onion, coarsely chopped

Combine the following and add: **½ cup vinegar**
1 tablespoon cornstarch
2 tablespoons brown sugar
1 tablespoon soy sauce
½ teaspoon ground ginger

Cook stirring constantly until thickened and then add:

1 can pineapple chunks and juice (19 ounces)

Arrange in a shallow baking dish: **1½ pounds fish fillets (sole, haddock, doré)**
salt lightly

Pour sweet and pungent sauce over the fish and bake in 350° oven for 30 minutes. Vegetable-fried rice goes very well with this.

VEGETABLE-BAKED FISH

Place: **2 pounds fish fillets or slices**

in a single layer in a large, shallow baking dish.

Over the fish place the following: **1 cup onion, chopped**
½ cup celery, chopped
½ cup fresh parsley, chopped, or 2 tablespoons dried
1 cup carrots, thinly sliced

2 potatoes, sliced
salt and pepper to taste

Spread over this: 1 can whole tomatoes (19 ounces)

Bake in 375° oven 45-60 minutes, or until fish is flaky and sauce bubbly. Baste frequently.

BARBECUED FISH FILLETS

Marinate: **1 pound fish fillets**

in the following sauce for 15 minutes each side.

Sauce

Combine: **¼ cup oil**
½ cup lemon juice
½ teaspoon salt
½ teaspoon black pepper
2 teaspoons instant minced onion
1 teaspoon dry mustard
2 tablespoons brown sugar

Broil the fillets 8 minutes on one side, turn, baste, and broil 5 minutes on the other side. The fish is done when it flakes easily.

TOMATO-TOPPED HADDOCK

Cut into serving
pieces: **1½ pounds fresh or frozen haddock fillets**

In skillet heat: **2 tablespoons oil**

Add: **1 medium onion, sliced thinly**
1 cup fresh mushrooms, sliced
1 small clove garlic, crushed

Cook gently about 3 minutes. Lay the pieces of fish on top of these vegetables.

Sprinkle with: **1 teaspoon salt**
¼ teaspoon crushed dill weed

Add: **1 20-ounce can tomatoes**

Partially cover and simmer for about 30 minutes (until fish flakes easily with a fork). Lift fish pieces out gently and place on a hot platter.

Blend until smooth: **1½ tablespoons flour**
2 tablespoons lemon juice

Add to hot mixture in the skillet, stirring constantly, bring to a boil and boil one minute. Pour the tomato sauce over the fish and sprinkle with parsley.

BROILED FISH WITH LEMON MUSTARD

Combine:
- ¼ cup lemon juice
- ¼ cup oil
- 1 tablespoon chopped parsley
- 2 teaspoons prepared mustard
- 1 teaspoon grated lemon rind
- ½ teaspoon salt
- ⅛ teaspoon pepper

On an oiled pan place: 1½ pounds of fish fillets

Brush with lemon mixture a few times while broiling. Broil about 10 minutes or until fish flakes easily with a fork. Do not turn. Serve immediately with lemon wedges.

BROILED HALIBUT STEAKS

Sprinkle: 4 halibut steaks
With:
- oil
- ¼ teaspoon garlic salt
- paprika
- salt and pepper to taste

Broil 10 minutes on each side or until fish flakes easily.

BAKED HALIBUT CREOLE

In a saucepan sauté:
- 1 onion, chopped
- 1 green pepper, diced
- 1 stalk celery, diced
- ½ pound mushrooms, sliced

Combine the following and add:
- 1 cup canned tomatoes
- ¼ teaspoon thyme
- ½ teaspoon basil
- ¼ teaspoon oregano
- salt and pepper to taste

Simmer covered for 5 minutes.

Then place: 1½ pounds halibut steaks

in a baking dish. Pour the vegetable mixture over the fish. Cover and bake in 350° oven for ½ hour. Uncover and bake 15 minutes longer.

SEAFOOD IN SHELLS

In a large skillet heat: 4 tablespoons oil

Add and cook for 4 minutes, stirring occasionally:

½ cup scallops cut into bite-sized pieces

½ cup canned or fresh crabmeat, flaked
½ cup raw shrimp cut into bite-sized pieces
2 tablespoons finely chopped onion

Sprinkle the
seafood mixture
with:

2 tablespoons sherry
½ teaspoon salt
¼ teaspoon freshly ground black pepper

In a saucepan
heat:

3 tablespoons oil

Add:

3 tablespoons flour

Stir until well blended. Bring to a boil and add to the flour mixture:

1½ cups skim milk

Stir vigorously until the sauce is thickened and smooth. Add the seafood mixture and spoon the mixture into 4 lightly oiled shells.

Sprinkle with: ⅓ cup bread crumbs

Bake in a 400° oven 12-15 minutes. Serve hot, garnished with lemon wedges.

COQUILLES ST. JACQUES

Sauté in oil
4-5 minutes:

1 pound scallops, cut in pieces
2 onions, chopped
½ pound mushrooms, sliced
2 cloves garlic, crushed

Combine the
following:

2 tablespoons flour
1 cup white wine
3 tablespoons chopped parsley
¼ teaspoon thyme
¼ teaspoon basil
salt and pepper to taste

Add the wine mixture to the scallops stirring steadily. Reduce heat and cook for 10 minutes.

Then add: ½ cup skim milk

Stir for 1 minute. *Do not boil.*

Fill shells or pie plate with scallops. Top with a mixture of:

¼ cup bread crumbs
2 tablespoons oil

Bake in 350° oven for 20 minutes. This makes 4-6 shells or fills one small pie plate.

BAKED ITALIAN SHRIMP OR FILLET

Heat: 2 tablespoons oil

Add: 1 clove garlic, crushed

Stir for 2 minutes and then add:	1 can Italian tomatoes (28 ounces)
	⅓ cup celery, chopped
	1 green pepper, chopped
	2 tablespoons parsley, chopped
	1 teaspoon salt
	¼ teaspoon pepper
	¼ teaspoon tarragon

Bring this to a boil. Cover and simmer for 30 minutes.

Shell, devein, and dry:	2 pounds shrimp (or fish fillets cut into shrimp-sized pieces)

Preheat oven to 450°. Put the tomato mixture in a large Pyrex baking dish and lay the shrimp over it in a single layer. Sprinkle the topping over the shrimp carefully and bake 20-25 minutes. Serve over plain white rice.

Topping

Combine:	½ cup Italian seasoned bread crumbs
	1 tablespoon parsley, chopped
	¼ cup oil

SALMON WITH ZUCCHINI AND CARROTS

Season:	1 pound salmon steaks
with:	salt
	pepper
Heat in a skillet:	2 tablespoons oil

Add salmon to pan and brown on both sides.

Add:	2 tablespoons lemon juice
	2 zucchini, sliced
	1 carrot, sliced very thin

Lower heat, cover skillet and cook for about 30-35 minutes.

POACHED SALMON

Bring to a boil:	1 quart water
	1 teaspoon salt
	1 onion
	1 carrot
	1 bay leaf
	a few peppercorns
	1 stalk of celery
	¼ cup vinegar

Reduce heat and simmer for about 15 minutes. Then add very gently:

a piece of salmon of desired size

If you are using a fairly large piece of salmon, wrap it in a piece of cheesecloth or a J cloth so that it can be removed easily after it is cooked. Simmer the salmon until tender—about 20 minutes. Remove the salmon carefully from the water, drain thoroughly and chill. Garnish with radish roses, sliced cucumber, and lemon slices. This is delicious served with the Mayonnaise Mustard Dressing.

SALMON STEAKS IN WINE

Dredge: **4 salmon steaks**

in: **flour**

Heat in a skillet: **2 tablespoons oil**

Fry the salmon until lightly browned. Remove the fish from the pan. Add the following to the pan and stir well for 1 minute:

> **½ cup dry white wine**
> **1 bay leaf**
> **1 tablespoon chopped parsley**
> **pinch of celery salt**
> **salt and pepper to taste**

Return steaks to the pan. Simmer covered for about 30 minutes or until fish flakes easily. Baste occasionally. Serve hot, and garnish with fresh parsley.

SALMON PATTIES

Drain, remove skin and bones from:

> **1 pound can of salmon**

Mash salmon   **1 small onion, grated**
and add: **1 small carrot, grated**
               1 egg (less half a yolk)
               1 tablespoon flour
               ¼ teaspoon baking powder
               salt and pepper to taste

Mix together and shape into patties.

Heat: **3 tablespoons oil**

Brown patties on both sides. Drain on absorbent paper. Serve with mashed potatoes and a vegetable for a nourishing hot lunch. These patties are delicious cold the next day.

PICKLED SALMON

The fish should be marinated in a *glass* dish or bowl.

Marinate   **4 medium slices of raw salmon**
overnight: **¼ cup sugar**

¾ cup vinegar
½ cup water
1 teaspoon mixed spices
1 teaspoon salt

Place fish in a large, shallow pan.

Add: **1 large Spanish onion, cut in ½-inch slices**

Pour marinade over fish and simmer half an hour, basting frequently. Refrigerate before serving. This will keep for 10 days in the refrigerator.

FISH ROLLS

Drain, remove skin and bones from:

1 8-ounce can salmon

Mash salmon   **1 teaspoon grated onion**
and add: **1 egg (less half yolk)**
                  2 tablespoons flour
                  salt and pepper to taste

Spread salmon mixture on:

6 pieces of raw fillet of sole

Roll as for jelly roll. Secure with white toothpicks. Place in baking pan and sprinkle a little oil on top. Bake in 350° oven until cooked—about half an hour. This goes well served with our Spanish Sauce. These rolls can be frozen raw, but remember to thaw before cooking.

TUNA-ASPARAGUS BAKE

In a small saucepan cook until golden:

2 tablespoons flour
1 tablespoon oil

Add, stirring until smooth:
1 cup hot skim milk

Then add: **1½ teaspoons grated onion**
                  ½ teaspoon dry mustard
                  1 teaspoon salt
                  1 tablespoon fresh or dried parsley, chopped

Cook over low heat until smooth and thickened.

In a one-quart casserole arrange:

1 can drained asparagus (fresh or frozen may be used)
1 can tuna rinsed with boiling water

Pour sauce over this and bake covered 15 minutes in 400° oven. Remove cover and let top brown slightly.

SPANISH SAUCE

Sauté until golden: **1 large onion, chopped, in**
1 tablespoon oil

Add: **½ green pepper, cut into strips**
1 stalk celery, sliced

Simmer covered for about 5 minutes, then add:

½ pound mushrooms, sliced
½ cup carrots, diced and cooked
1 small zucchini, diced and cooked

Stir and cook until mushrooms are tender.

Then add: **2 cans tomato sauce (8 ounces)**

to which has been added:

1 tablespoon flour

Season to taste
with: **salt**
pepper
pinch of sugar

Continue simmering until sauce is slightly thickened. This sauce freezes very well. Make up a batch and have some on hand for any plain boiled or broiled fish.

ALMOND-ORANGE SAUCE

In a skillet heat: **2 tablespoons oil**

Sauté until golden brown:

2 tablespoons blanched almonds

Remove the almonds.

Combine: **1½ tablespoons brown sugar**
2 teaspoons cornstarch
1 cup orange juice

Then add to same skillet and cook over medium heat stirring constantly until clear and thickened.

Add: **1½ tablespoons grated orange rind**
¼ teaspoon powdered cloves (optional)
½ teaspoon seasoned salt
the browned almonds

Serve hot over broiled fish.

Chapter 17 • Vegetables

Vegetables should be an essential part of any daily menu. They are nutritious and, if prepared well, are most delicious. For purposes of fat control, you should serve larger portions of vegetables and will then need smaller portions of meat to round out a meal.

The key word in good vegetables is *fresh;* the fresher the vegetables are, the better they will taste. No amount of preparation will improve an old vegetable.

The best, easiest, and most healthful way to prepare vegetables is by steaming them. An investment in a steamer will pay high dividends. A small amount of water goes under the steamer and the vegetables sit on the rack. In this way, the vitamins aren't washed out into the water you throw away, but stay in the vegetables. In steaming, as well as in any other preparation, never overcook vegetables—it diminishes nutritional value as well as flavor.

Use Oil Instead

Whenever possible, we try to replace fat or butter with more healthful ingredients. Oil can easily replace the butter used in many vegetable dishes. When preparing sautéed vegetables, such as mushrooms, onions, and Chinese vegetables, use oil rather than butter in your pan. Did you know that you can brown mushrooms, onions, and other vegetables in a pan prepared without oil or butter? You can now buy a spray-on coating that will prepare your pan. If you desire, when the onions start to brown you can add water and simmer without loss of flavor. This will give you a good base for cooking.

Instead of topping your vegetables with butter, use a little oil and add a generous shake of your favorite seasoning. If you are lucky enough to be able to buy farm-fresh vegetables, you will quickly discover that you can enjoy their fresh flavor with nothing added.

Many people are in the habit of smothering their potatoes with butter. A healthful alternative is to prepare mashed potatoes adding a little oil and a little skim milk so they will have a rich flavor. Rubbing oil on the skins of baked potatoes before baking will help keep the skins soft. Then, when serving, use some of our "sour cream" instead of butter. (The recipe can be found in chapter 12.) The "sour cream" can be garnished with chopped chives or bacon substitute to provide a four-star restaurant effect.

Seasoning

For that little extra something for your vegetables, look to your spice shelf. Following are some of the combinations that we have found enticing:

Suggested Seasonings	Vegetables
Curry powder	zucchini cabbage carrots
Dried basil	carrots yellow squash beans tomatoes
Nutmeg	turnips beans peas
Dried mustard	beans spinach broccoli
Chopped parsley	corn cauliflower potatoes cabbage
Rosemary	peas cauliflower squash
Ginger	carrots Chinese types of vegetables

DUTCH GREEN BEANS

Cook together and
set aside:

1 package frozen green beans
1 medium onion, sliced

Combine, then bring to a boil stirring constantly:

⅓ cup water
⅓ cup vinegar

> 1 teaspoon cornstarch
> ¼ cup brown sugar

Drain cooked beans, add sauce, and simmer 2 minutes longer. Serve hot.

HARVARD BEETS

Combine the following and cook until clear and thickened, stirring constantly:

> ½ cup sugar
> ½ tablespoon cornstarch
> ¼ cup vinegar
> ¼ cup juice from 1 can of beets

Then add: 1 can diced beets (drained)

Mix until the beets are well coated with the sauce. Keep warm until time to serve.

BROCCOLI WITH BREAD CRUMBS

Cook or steam as usual:

> 1 pound fresh or 1 package frozen broccoli

Brown: ½ cup seasoned bread crumbs in
2 tablespoons oil

Add: 1 teaspoon chopped parsley

Mix well and sprinkle over cooked broccoli on the serving platter. Cauliflower may be substituted for broccoli.

BOILED CARROTS

Cook until tender: 6 unpeeled young carrots
1 teaspoon salt

Gently remove skins under running water. Slice 1-inch thick pieces on the diagonal and return to the pan.

Add: 2 teaspoons oil
salt to taste
a few shakes of fresh ground pepper

Serve hot. Carrots have an unusual flavor when cooked this way.

CANDIED CARROTS

Cut into strips and boil until tender in salted water:

> 6 carrots

Drain and arrange in baking dish. Combine and heat until sugar is dissolved:

> ⅓ cup water
> ⅓ cup brown sugar
> 2 teaspoons oil

Pour the syrup over the carrots and bake in 350° oven for 45 minutes. Baste occasionally.

CARROTS AND PEPPERS

Boil until tender in salted water:

> 4 carrots, sliced on the diagonal
> ½ teaspoon dried basil

Meanwhile, sauté in a skillet:

> 1 tablespoon oil
> 3 tablespoons minced green peppers

Toss together and serve hot.

CARROT PUDDING

Combine in large mixing bowl:

> ½ cup oil
> ½ cup brown sugar
> 1 egg
> 1 tablespoon water

Add:

> 1½ cups sifted all-purpose flour
> 1 teaspoon baking powder
> ½ teaspoon salt
> ½ teaspoon baking soda
> ½ teaspoon cinnamon
> ½ teaspoon nutmeg
> 4 cups grated carrots (about 8 medium)

(For speed, cut carrots may be put through fine blade of meat grinder.) Pour into oiled ovenproof serving dish. Refrigerate overnight. Remove about an hour before baking and bake in 350° oven for one hour. If your baking dish is small and deep, allow a little more baking time.

CORN ALMANDINE

Brown lightly in a saucepan:

> 1 tablespoon oil
> 3 tablespoons slivered almonds

Then stir in:

> 1 12-ounce can of whole-kernel corn, well drained

Serve hot.

CORN FRITTERS

Prepare a batter of:

> ½ cup skim milk
> 1 tablespoon oil

                1 cup flour
                1 teaspoon baking powder
                1 egg
                ¼ teaspoon salt
                pepper

Add: **1½ cups corn kernels, fresh or canned**

Heat: **3 tablespoons oil**

Drop batter into the oil by the spoonful. Fry until golden, about 3-4 minutes on each side. Drain on paper towels. To keep hot, arrange fritters on a cookie sheet in a single layer and place in a warm oven.

FRUIT FRITTERS

Combine: **½ cup skim milk**
                1 tablespoon oil
                1 cup flour
                1 teaspoon baking powder
                2 tablespoons sugar
                pinch salt
                1 egg

Prepare thin slices of any of the following:

                apples
                pineapple
                bananas, sliced lengthwise

Dip in batter, and fry until golden on both sides in:

                oil

Drain on paper towels. To keep hot, arrange fritters on a cookie sheet in a single layer and place in a warm oven. Sprinkle with powdered sugar and serve garnished with lemon wedges.

BAKED EGGPLANT CASSEROLE

Prepare: **1 eggplant cut in ¼-inch slices (peeled or unpeeled)**
                4 medium tomatoes, sliced
                2 green peppers, thinly sliced
                2 onions, sliced

Combine: **1 tablespoon sugar**
                1 teaspoon salt
                ¼ teaspoon pepper
                ½ teaspoon garlic salt

In a lightly oiled 2-quart casserole, place a layer of eggplant, add a layer of tomatoes, then a layer of the green pepper and onion slices. Sprinkle lightly with seasonings. Repeat until the casserole is heaped high. The vegetables will shrink during cooking. Sprinkle with:

Italian seasoned bread crumbs

Cover the casserole and bake in a 400° oven for 30 minutes. Remove the cover, reduce the heat to 350° and continue cooking 45 minutes longer. Serve piping hot.

RATATOUILLE

In a large saucepan heat:

        4 tablespoons oil

Add: **2 medium onions, sliced**
        2 green or red peppers cut into fine strips
        1 clove garlic, crushed
        1 teaspoon salt

Cover, cook gently for 15 minutes—do not allow onion to brown.

Peel and cut: **1 medium eggplant into cubes (1-1½ pounds)**
        1 pound zucchini into ¼-inch slices

Add eggplant and zucchini to onion mixture. Cover and cook gently for 30 minutes.

Add: **1 pound tomatoes peeled and coarsely chopped**
        1 teaspoon sugar
        1 tablespoon chopped parsley
        black pepper

Re-cover and cook 15 minutes longer, or until vegetables are tender. This unusual combination makes just as big a hit whether served cold or hot.

RICE AND NOODLES

Sauté until golden: **¼ cup oil**
        1 small onion finely cut

Add: **2 cups of "5-minute rice"**
        2 cups of raw fine noodles

Continue stirring until brown.

Then add: **3⅓ cups boiling chicken stock**
        1 teaspoon salt
        pepper

Bring to a boil. Remove from heat and allow to stand five minutes.

NOODLES AND NOODLES

Boil until tender in salted water and set aside:

        1½ cups broad noodles

Sauté until golden: **1 small onion very finely chopped**
        2 tablespoons oil

Add: ½ cup fine raw noodles slightly crushed (1-inch pieces)

Continue cooking, stirring constantly until noodles are brown. Add drained broad noodles, toss together, season to taste with:

salt
pepper
½ teaspoon instant chicken soup powder

Serve hot in place of potatoes.

PEAS AND ONIONS

Drain, reserving juice, and set aside:

1 14-ounce can of peas

To the juice add: 1 sliced onion
1½ teaspoons sugar

Simmer until tender, about 20 minutes.

Then add: 1 tablespoon flour

Simmer for a few more minutes.

Add: peas

Heat through and serve.

MINTED GREEN PEAS

Cook as directed: 1 package frozen peas

with: 2 teaspoons minced onions
1 teaspoon dried mint leaves

Drain and toss
with: 2 teaspoons oil

Serve hot.

GREEN PEAS ITALIANO

Combine in a   1 pound green peas, shelled
saucepan: ¾ cup uncooked rice (not instant)
1 carrot, diced
pinch of thyme
¼ teaspoon basil
½ teaspoon sugar
1 teaspoon salt

Then add: 2 cups water, consommé, or milk

Bring to a boil over medium heat, stirring once or twice. Lower heat, cover, and simmer 20 minutes or until the peas are tender and the rice has absorbed all the liquid. Place in a heated vegetable dish and sprinkle with minced parsley.

SCALLOPED POTATOES

Lightly oil a baking dish and arrange in layers:

5 medium potatoes pared and thinly sliced

Dredge the layers with flour, salt, and pepper. Use in all:

**2 tablespoons flour
salt and pepper to taste**

Pour over this: **1¼ cups hot skim milk**

Blend together: **2 tablespoons bread crumbs
1 tablespoon grated skim milk cheese
1 teaspoon oil
a few shakes of paprika**

Sprinkle over potatoes and bake in a 350° oven for about one hour or until potatoes are cooked.

POTATO PANCAKES OR PUDDINGS

Grate on fine side of grater into a bowl of cold water:

6 medium potatoes

Drain the potatoes well and then add: **1 small onion, grated
4 tablespoons flour
1 teaspoon baking powder
1½ teaspoons salt
pepper
1 egg**

In a skillet heat: **3 tablespoons oil**

Drop potato mixture by the spoonful into the hot oil and flatten out. When brown, turn and fry on other side. Drain on paper towels. To keep hot, arrange in single layer on cookie sheet and put in warm oven.

To make small potato puddings, put a half teaspoon of oil in muffin pans and fill each pan half full with the potato mixture. Bake in 400° oven 30-45 minutes until brown. Serve hot. These freeze very well if you have any left over!

MASHED POTATOES

Boil in salted water until tender:

6 potatoes (peeled and cut into pieces)

Mash the potatoes **salt**
and then add: **pepper**
1 tablespoon oil
skim milk (to desired consistency)

Beat until light and fluffy. Serve piping hot.

ONION-MASHED POTATOES

In a large saucepan fry until very brown, nearly burnt:

2 medium onions, chopped fine, in
1½ tablespoons oil

Add: **6 medium potatoes peeled and cut into small pieces**
salt, pepper, and paprika to taste
water enough to cover potatoes

Cook partially covered until potatoes are very soft. Mash without draining water (water should be nearly all evaporated). You won't believe how good this is.

OVEN-ROASTED POTATOES

Peel and cut into ½-inch slices:

2-3 medium potatoes (Idaho preferred)

Blot them dry with paper toweling, and rub each potato piece with:

oil

Sprinkle with: **salt**
pepper
paprika
garlic salt (optional)

Place on a flat cookie sheet and bake in a 400° oven until tender and golden (for 30-45 minutes).

BOILED NEW POTATOES

Boil until cooked, without peeling:

small new potatoes

Drain, peel, and **salt**
add: **freshly ground pepper**
oil
chopped parsley

Serve hot. We enjoy eating these hot potatoes served with cold "sour cream" (see recipe).

STUFFED BAKED POTATOES VANCOUVER

Wash and dry: **6 medium baking potatoes**

Bake for 1 hour or until fork tender in a 400° oven. Cut a slice from the top of each potato, remove potato leaving shell.

In a bowl beat
together:
- **potato**
- **2 tablespoons oil**
- **½ cup warm skim milk**
- **1 egg, less half the yolk**
- **2 teaspoons salt**
- **¼ teaspoon pepper**

Refill the shells and sprinkle with:

oil

paprika

Bake the potatoes in 400° oven for about 15 minutes. These potatoes are delicious served with "sour cream" (see recipe) or sprinkle with chives.

After refilling the shells, the potatoes can be cooled and then wrapped for the freezer and frozen for up to one month. Thaw before baking.

PAN-FRIED POTATOES

Peel, shred coarsely, or cut very fine:

4 large potatoes

Pat dry in a clean towel. In a heavy pan heat over medium-high heat:

¼ cup oil

Add:
- **prepared potatoes**
- **½ teaspoon salt**
- **pepper**
- **paprika**
- **onion powder**

Reduce heat to medium. Allow potatoes to cook uncovered, for about half an hour or until potatoes are cooked and brown. Stir occasionally. Serve hot and make lots.

SWEET POTATO AND CARROT TZIMMES

Parboil: **1 pound carrots (½-inch slices)**

Place in a
casserole:
- **parboiled carrots**
- **2 pounds sweet potatoes, peeled and cut into 1-inch pieces**
- **1 pound pitted prunes**
- **10 diced, dried apricot halves cut into small pieces**
- **some very small pieces of lean meat (optional)**

Combine the following and pour over the above:

> ¾ cup orange juice
> juice and rind of half a lemon
> 1 or 2 tablespoons orange marmalade
> 2 tablespoons brown sugar
> 1 teaspoon salt

Bake covered in 350° oven for 1½ hours, and then uncovered for an additional hour. Without meat, cook for only 2 hours.

JAVANESE FRIED RICE

This rice cooks twice. It takes a little extra time to prepare, but is well worth the effort.

Boil:
> 4 cups water
> 2 bouillon cubes
> ½ teaspoon curry powder
> 1 teaspoon salt

Add:
> 2 cups uncooked rice

Cover and cook 15-20 minutes (until the liquid is absorbed). Chill the rice. The rice should be dry and the grains separate before frying.

Sauté until golden:
> 1 large chopped onion
> 1 clove minced garlic
> 1 tablespoon oil

Remove onions and garlic and set aside. Fluff the rice with fork to separate. Sauté the rice lightly, doing only ½ at a time. For each batch use:

> 2 tablespoons oil

Then return all the rice to the pan, and add:
> onions and garlic that have been set aside
> ½ teaspoon chili powder
> ¼ teaspoon mace
> ½ cup toasted slivered almonds

Cover and heat slowly. Serve hot.

VEGETABLE FRIED RICE

Sauté until golden:
> 3 tablespoons oil
> 2 medium onions, chopped fine
> 2 stalks celery, sliced
> ½ green pepper, chopped
> salt and pepper

Add:
> 1 package mushrooms, sliced
> 1 small jar chopped pimentoes

When this mixture is cooked add:

> 1½ cups water
> 4 tablespoons soy sauce

Bring to a rapid boil, then remove from heat and add:

2 cups instant rice

Cover and let stand five minutes. A chopped tomato may be added just as the water boils, before adding rice. The cooked vegetables may be prepared ahead of time and frozen in small amounts. Three tablespoons of cooked vegetables, plus ¾ cup water, 2 teaspoons soy sauce and ¾ cup instant rice will serve 2 people.

SPANISH RICE

Fry together until rice is brown:

2 tablespoons oil
¾ cup rice

Add and simmer covered until tender:

1¾ cups salted water

Sauté until golden: **2 small onions, chopped**
½ cup green pepper, chopped
salt and pepper

Add to this: **2 cups canned whole tomatoes**

Mix together with rice. Place in lightly oiled baking dish and bake in 350° oven for 30 minutes.

CREAMED SPINACH

Cook as directed: **1 package frozen chopped spinach**

Drain, reserving liquid and set aside. Combine and cook over medium heat until bubbly:

1 tablespoon flour
1 tablespoon oil

Then add slowly: **⅓ cup skim milk powder added to reserved liquid and enough water to make 1 cup**

Cook slowly until thick and smooth. Add drained spinach and season well with:

salt
pepper
garlic salt
ground nutmeg

Serve hot.

BAKED STUFFED TOMATOES

Cut off tops of: **4 medium tomatoes**

Scoop out centers, chop pulp, and combine with:

>**2 tablespoons minced green pepper**
>**1 tablespoon minced onion**
>**¼ teaspoon salt**
>**dash of pepper**

Place tomato mixture back into shells.

In another dish blend:
>**2 tablespoons oil**
>**¼ cup fine bread crumbs**

Spoon the crumbs on top of the tomatoes. Place in shallow baking dish in 375° oven for 15-20 minutes. Serve hot.

SKILLET ZUCCHINI

Wash, peel if desired, cut into 1-inch slices, and set aside:

>**4 medium zucchini (about 1 pound)**

Heat in skillet:
>**2 tablespoons oil**

Sauté:
>**1 onion, sliced**

until lightly browned.

Then add:
>**2 fresh tomatoes, peeled and chopped**
>**1 tablespoon pimento, chopped**
>**1 teaspoon salt**
>**¼ teaspoon pepper**
>**1 bay leaf**
>**½ teaspoon crushed basil**

Cover and cook 5 minutes. Add the zucchini. Cover and simmer for about 20 minutes longer, or until the zucchini is tender. This is an attractive dish as well as delicious.

MIXED VEGETABLE CASSEROLE

Cook until nearly tender:

>**1 package mixed frozen vegetables**

Prepare and add:
>**½ cup of "cream sauce" (see recipe)**
>**1 teaspoon instant mushroom or chicken soup**

Gently add:
>**drained vegetables**

and place in a casserole. Cover with a mixture of:

>**1 cup dry cereal crushed (unsweetened type)**
>**1 tablespoon oil**
>**½ teaspoon onion powder**

Bake in a 350° oven until top is lightly browned, about 30 minutes. Serve hot. Any other cooked vegetables can be substituted.

Chapter 18 • Salads

Salads can be served as a first course, a main course, or as an accompanying dish. They can be based on meat, poultry, fish, vegetables, or fruit. The combinations are endless—just allow your imagination full rein.

First Course

Get into the habit of enjoying large servings of salad at the beginning of a meal to take the sharp edge off an unruly appetite. In addition to a tossed salad, try something a little more distinctive such as a tomato stuffed with corn, or slices of cucumber and tomatoes with Italian dressing. From one of our favorite restaurants we got the idea of combining crabmeat and grapefruit served in the grapefruit shell—it is delicious.

Main Course

Some salads are strong enough to stand on their own; attractive combinations using fish or poultry as a base can be served as the whole meal. Salade Niçoise or Party Chicken Salad are two suggestions that you will find in the recipe section.

Try new combinations. For example, cold chicken can be combined with pineapple, nuts, grapes, or rice. Remember, each new combination is a new meal. A large tossed salad made with cubes of lean meat, such as flank steak or ham, and a mustard dressing is absolutely delicious. Serve with a crisp, fresh roll or French bread for a complete meal.

Fruit salads are always refreshing and are especially enjoyable in summer when there is such a large variety of fresh fruit available. Any combination of fruit served on crisp lettuce, accompanied by cottage cheese, yogurt, flavored gelatin, and a warm, fresh roll makes a delicious lunch or even dinner on a hot day.

Accompanying Dishes

The most traditional way to serve salad is as an accompanying dish. We often think of vegetable salads accompanying a meal, but fruit may also be served, either alone or combined with the vegetables.

If the scheduled meal for a Sunday barbecue is hamburgers, it is likely that you would eat two or more. However, with a large salad, you could easily keep this down to one, thereby having an enjoyable meal but not pushing your fat consumption up to unacceptable levels.

Do It Right

Since greens are the main ingredient of many salads, learn how to care for them so that they will always be as tasty and as appetizing as possible. To be served at their peak, salad greens must be crisp, dry, and cool. The best way we have found is to wash and dry the lettuce, wrap it in a clean towel, and then place it in the vegetable crisper of the refrigerator for a few hours.

Variety Is Important

Why use the same type of lettuce all the time when there are so many types available? Vary your salads with Boston lettuce, escarole, endive, or spinach greens. Grated cabbage for a coleslaw makes a nice change.

Mixed green salad can be changed into a hundred different salads with a little imagination. Remember, you are trying to replace some of the unwanted foods with increased salad intake, so think of pleasant combinations with good contrasts in both color and flavor. Make your salad pleasing to the eye, with attractive garnishes such as radish roses, thin carrot strips, pimento, snips of anchovies, or raw mushrooms.

Salad Dressings

Remember to choose your salad dressing carefully to be certain it complements the salad. The same vegetables with a different dressing will often taste like a different salad.

Oil-based dressings are preferable to the mayonnaise types. If you use the latter, however, always use the salad dressing type of mayonnaise since it contains less egg yolk than pure mayonnaise. The most suitable types of dressings to use are the ones in which you combine your own oil and vinegar. We have a large selection of dressing recipes in this book, so there is no need to buy prepared ones.

The addition of herbs creates a variety of taste delights. Many of our recipes show you specifically how to make use of these. In the summer we grow some of our own herbs, which are so much better than the jar variety. They take only a little space to grow and can even be grown indoors—so why not try growing a herb garden of your own?

It is important to keep the salad aspects of menu planning in perspective. Anyone who has gone on a simple weight-reducing diet will remember eating lots of salads (usually too many) and is probably left with an unenthusiastic attitude toward them. This need not be so. For our purposes, salads should be used with a different goal in mind. We are trying to change the overall *balance* of the menu. We are not giving up good food to eat only lettuce and tomatoes; we are stressing the importance of eating salads to diminish, but not abolish, consumption of meat.

For example, an attractive salad served with supper might mean that a four-ounce serving of meat becomes as filling a meal as a six-ounce serving might otherwise be. This is a significant saving, but unlike old-fashioned dieting, the eater has not starved himself by eating only salad for supper.

Similarly, when making a weekend lunch, a little extra time taken to garnish a chicken salad attractively will produce a filling meal that need not be thought of as "just a salad." Other salads can be served with sandwiches or soup to make a more varied meal. The idea is to put thought into salad planning to insure that your family successfully uses this method of eating the amount of food they need, while cutting down on meat and fats.

TUNA MACARONI SALAD

Cook:	½ pound of shell macaroni

Drain the macaroni, rinse with cold water, and drain again.

To the macaroni, add:	⅓ cup mayonnaise (salad dressing type)
	1 tablespoon chopped onion

Cool and then add the following ingredients:	½ cup chopped celery
	¼ cup chopped green pepper
	1 can drained tuna
	1 teaspoon salt
	¼ teaspoon pepper

TUNA VERONIQUE

Combine:	1 7-ounce can of drained, flaked tuna
	½ cup green or red grapes, halved and seeded

½ cup chopped celery
2 tablespoons toasted, slivered almonds
⅛ teaspoon curry powder
3 tablespoons mayonnaise (salad dressing type)

Chill this for a few hours and serve as a salad base.

SEAFOOD SALAD

Mix together
lightly:

1 cup flaked, cooked seafood (crabmeat, tuna,
  salmon, lobster)
1 teaspoon lemon juice
1 teaspoon minced onion
salt and paprika to taste
1 cup diced celery

Just before serving, drain and moisten with:

mayonnaise (salad dressing type)

Serve on a bed of crisp lettuce and garnish with:

wedges of lemon
wedges of tomato

SALADE NIÇOISE

This is a marvelous salad for last-minute lunches when unexpected company comes over. Most of the ingredients can be stored on the pantry shelf.

In a large salad bowl place:

6-8 cups crisp salad greens in bite-sized pieces

Add:

2 7-ounce cans of white meat tuna (in chunks)
½ cup pitted ripe olives, drained
2 tablespoons capers, drained
2 tomatoes cut into quarters
1 small cucumber, peeled and thinly sliced
1 2-ounce can anchovy fillets, drained and sliced
1 green pepper cut into strips
1 small red onion, thinly sliced

Just before serving, toss well with a:

basic French dressing

If you want to chill the salad before serving, do so, but add the dressing *just* before serving.

PARTY CHICKEN SALAD

Toss together:

2 cups of cooked chicken, diced
1 cup chopped celery

1 tablespoon lemon juice
salt and pepper to taste

Add: ½ cup mayonnaise (salad dressing type)
1 cup drained pineapple chunks

Sprinkle with: ½ cup toasted, slivered almonds

Serve this on a crisp lettuce bed. Garnish with:

olives
tomato wedges

CHEF'S SALAD

Place in a salad bowl:

4-6 cups bite-sized pieces of crisp salad greens

Add: 2 tomatoes cut in wedges
1 apple cored and cut into very thin strips
1 green pepper cut into rings
4 radishes, sliced

Toss with sufficient:

French dressing

to coat the greens.

Arrange attractively on the salad:

1 cup cooked chicken breasts cut into julienne strips
½ cup lean ham cut into julienne strips

Garnish with: parsley

CHICKEN AND RICE SALAD

In a large bowl, 2 cups cooked rice
combine and set 2 cups cooked chicken, diced
aside: 1½ cups cooked peas
1½ cups celery, diced
1 tablespoon grated onion

Combine in ½ cup mayonnaise (salad dressing type)
another bowl: 1 teaspoon salt
¼ teaspoon pepper

Combine the mayonnaise mixture with the chicken mixture. Chill for at least an hour before serving.

Serve on: crisp salad greens

and garnish with: bright red tomato slices

MOLDED WALDORF SALAD

Dissolve: **1 3-ounce package of lemon or lime gelatin**

in: **1 cup boiling water**

Chill until slightly thickened.

Fold in: **1 cup finely diced apple**
                         ¼ cup thinly sliced celery
                         ¼ cup chopped pecans

Pour into individual molds. Chill until firm. When ready to use, unmold on:

                         crisp salad greens

This is very decorative as well as delicious.

CHICKEN SALAD MOLD

In a small saucepan, soften:

                         1 envelope unflavored gelatin

in: **1¼ cups pineapple juice**

Add: **½ teaspoon salt**

Heat and stir until the gelatin dissolves.

In a bowl,   **1 8-ounce container of lemon or pineapple yogurt**
combine: **2 tablespoons mayonnaise (salad dressing type)**

Stir the gelatin into the yogurt mixture and chill until partially set.

Fold in: **1½ cups cooked chicken, diced**
                         ¼ cup chopped celery
                         2 tablespoons toasted, slivered almonds

Pour into 6 individual ½ cup molds or 1 3-cup mold, and chill until firm.

Unmold onto: **lettuce cups**

Garnish with any of the following:

                         cherry tomatoes
                         clusters of grapes
                         parsley
                         cranberry relish or slices

SALMON-STUFFED TOMATOES

Mix thoroughly: **1 cup salmon (canned or fresh-poached)**
                         ⅓ cup mayonnaise (salad dressing type)
                         ½ tablespoon catsup
                         ½ teaspoon chopped chives
                         ¼ teaspoon tarragon

Cut the tops off of: **4 large ripe tomatoes (set the tops aside)**

Empty the tomato pulp with a small spoon. Season the interior of the tomatoes with salt and fill them with the salmon mixture. Put the top of the tomatoes back on and refrigerate until serving time. These are especially good served with asparagus.

WILTED CUCUMBERS

Peel and slice very thin:

**2 medium cucumbers
½ Spanish onion (optional)**

Place in ice water in refrigerator for half an hour.

Combine: **½ cup water
½ cup vinegar
1 teaspoon salt
2 tablespoons sugar**

Drain cucumbers well, add vinegar mixture, and refrigerate 3 or 4 hours.

Serve with: **a sprinkle of freshly ground pepper**

BASIL TOMATOES

Combine: **2 tablespoons oil
1 teaspoon vinegar
½ teaspoon dried or 1 teaspoon chopped fresh basil
salt and pepper to taste**

Slice thinly: **3 medium tomatoes**

Sprinkle each slice with the marinade. Cover and chill for at least two hours.

THREE-BEAN SALAD

Drain and place in a bowl: **1 16-ounce can red kidney beans
1 16-ounce can yellow wax beans or chick peas
1 16-ounce can French-cut green beans**

Add: **½ cup finely chopped green pepper
½ cup minced onion**

Combine in a jar: **½ cup oil
¼ cup cider vinegar
1 tablespoon sugar
1 teaspoon salt
½ teaspoon pepper**

Shake very well and then pour the oil mixture over the beans and toss, making sure the beans are well coated. Cover and chill for several hours before serving.

CARROT AND RAISIN SALAD

Combine thoroughly:	1 teaspoon sugar
	½ teaspoon salt
	3 tablespoons mayonnaise (salad dressing type)
	1 tablespoon lemon juice
Add:	3 medium carrots, shredded
	½ cup raisins

Toss lightly until thoroughly mixed. Allow to marinate a few hours or overnight before serving.

FROSTED GRAPES

Dip small clusters of:	seedless grapes
in:	1 egg white, slightly beaten

When they are nearly dry, sprinkle with:

granulated sugar

These are easy to prepare and they look so pretty as a garnish for poultry, meats, or molded salads.

MAYONNAISE I
Salad Dressing Type

Combine in a bowl:	½ teaspoon sugar
	½ teaspoon dry mustard
	¼ teaspoon salt
	dash red pepper
Add:	1 egg white

Beat well with a rotary beater. Beating constantly add a *little at a time:*

½ cup oil

Continue beating and add:	1½ teaspoons vinegar
Very slowly add another:	½ cup oil
Then add:	1 teaspoon lemon juice
	2 teaspoons vinegar

Continue beating until blended. Makes about 1 cup.

MAYONNAISE II
Salad Dressing Type

Beat at high speed of electric mixer until frothy:

              1 egg
              1 tablespoon lemon juice

Add: **1¼ teaspoons sugar**
              1 teaspoon salt
              1 teaspoon dry mustard
              ¼ teaspoon paprika

Beat well.

Add very slowly: **1 cup oil**

Continue beating slowly until the mixture becomes thick. When the mixture is very thick add:

              another tablespoon lemon juice
              1 tablespoon vinegar

Continue adding: **another cup of oil**

gradually until well blended, thick and creamy. This makes about 2 cups.

MAYONNAISE DRESSING

Combine: **⅔ cup mayonnaise (salad dressing type)**
              ⅓ cup vinegar
              ½ teaspoon salt
              ¼ teaspoon pepper
              2 teaspoons sugar
              ½ teaspoon dry mustard

Stir until completely blended.

THOUSAND ISLAND DRESSING

Combine: **2 cups mayonnaise (salad dressing type)**
              ¼ cup chili sauce
              ½ cup catsup
              1 teaspoon Worcestershire sauce
              1 teaspoon paprika
              ¼ cup sweet pickle relish
              ½ cup finely chopped green pepper
              1 teaspoon grated onion

Chill well before serving.

CURRY MAYONNAISE

Combine
thoroughly:

1 cup mayonnaise (salad dressing type)
1 teaspoon curry powder
juice of half a lemon

This dressing goes well with either chicken or shrimp.

HERB DRESSING

Combine in a jar:

1½ cups mayonnaise (salad dressing type)
1½ teaspoons prepared mustard
½ teaspoon Tabasco sauce
2 teaspoons chili powder
1 teaspoon onion juice
2 tablespoons vinegar
1½ teaspoons marjoram
¾ teaspoon thyme
1½ teaspoons minced garlic

Shake well before using.

MUSTARD MAYONNAISE DRESSING

Combine:

2 tablespoons mayonnaise (salad dressing type)
1 tablespoon prepared mustard
½ teaspoon lemon juice

Serve this with a cold fish salad.

TARTAR SAUCE

Chop and combine:

1 teaspoon stuffed olives
1 teaspoon capers
1 teaspoon sweet pickle
½ teaspoon chopped parsley

Add:

½ cup mayonnaise
½ teaspoon finely grated onion
1 teaspoon lemon juice

Place in a covered jar and refrigerate until ready to use.

LEMON DRESSING

Dissolve:

½ teaspoon sugar

in:

4 tablespoons lemon juice

Add:

¼ teaspoon salt
dash of pepper
4 tablespoons oil

Shake well and pour over the salad.

GARLIC DRESSING

Combine all
ingredients in
a jar:

½ cup oil
¼ cup wine vinegar
¼ teaspoon Worcestershire sauce
½ teaspoon prepared hot mustard
1 clove minced garlic
¾ teaspoon salt
freshly ground pepper

Refrigerate for several hours, and shake well before using.

BASIC FRENCH DRESSING

Combine all
ingredients in a
jar or bottle:

1 cup oil
⅓ cup vinegar
1 teaspoon sugar
1½ teaspoons salt
½ teaspoon paprika
½ teaspoon dry mustard
1 clove garlic (optional)

Cover jar tightly and shake well. Chill several hours, then remove garlic.
Shake thoroughly before serving.

GOLDEN FRENCH DRESSING

Combine
ingredients in a
jar or bottle:

2 teaspoons prepared mustard
2 teaspoons salt
1 teaspoon sugar
few grains pepper
1 teaspoon Worcestershire sauce
½ cup vinegar
1 cup oil
1 clove minced garlic (optional)

Cover tightly and shake well. Refrigerate for several hours and shake
thoroughly before serving.

REAL ITALIAN DRESSING

Measure into a jar
or bottle and
shake well:

⅔ cup oil
3 tablespoons wine vinegar
1 tablespoon water
1 teaspoon salt
2 teaspoons sugar
1½ teaspoons lemon juice
¼ teaspoon garlic powder

dash red pepper
dash oregano

Chill for several hours and shake well before using.

HONEY-YOGURT DRESSING

Combine:
1 cup skim milk yogurt
½ cup pineapple juice
2 tablespoons honey
½ teaspoon salt

This dressing is especially good for fruit salads.

COTTAGE CHEESE DRESSING

Combine until
creamy:
6 ounces cottage cheese
½ cup pineapple juice
¼ cup lemon juice
drop of red food coloring

Mix thoroughly and chill well. This is a very good dressing for fruit salads.

Chapter 19 • Baking

Everybody enjoys cakes and cookies and misses them on a diet. In our plan, you are actually encouraged to eat baked goodies and we have a special reason for this. As we explained before, it is important not only to decrease your saturated fat, but also to increase your unsaturated fat intake. One of the most pleasant ways to do this is by eating homemade desserts.

Most of the products in your local bakery or pastry shop contain too much saturated fat. Nearly all of the same baked goods can be made with unsaturated fat; we have included a large list of easy and delicious recipes in this category to provide the desserts your family loves to eat.

Revising Your Own Recipes

Many of the recipes in this book have been adapted from old favorites, substituting unsaturated for saturated fats. You can use some of your own favorites in the same way. When you bake cakes that contain three or four eggs, omit one yolk and add two additional teaspoons of oil. Next time try leaving out another yolk. Now you will be using only two yolks in a four-egg cake. We have been able to devise recipes for sponge and chiffon cakes that call for only a few egg yolks. These cakes are as light as those made with a greater number of whole eggs, and can be garnished in many ways to provide a variety of desserts.

Another ingredient that can easily be substituted is baking chocolate. For each square of chocolate required, use two tablespoons of unsweetened cocoa plus one tablespoon of oil. Chocolate is cocoa plus cocoa butter, so by substituting the oil, you are replacing most of the saturated fat with unsaturated fat.

Remember that because of its very high saturated fat content, coconut is absolutely forbidden. If your family is very fond of it, artificial coconut flavoring is available.

If any of your refrigerator-gelatin desserts call for whipped cream as an ingredient, try the following substitute. For each cup of whipped cream needed use:

¾ cup skim milk powder
¾ cup ice water
4 teaspoons lemon juice

Whip until very stiff—for at least eight minutes. When preparing the gelatin part of the dessert, add an additional half package of gelatin for each cup of whipped cream called for. You will be amazed at the results.

Oil is the only fat used in our recipes. Recipes that call for a large amount of butter or shortening may not always turn out exactly the same when you substitute oil. You can achieve excellent results, however, by experimentation and slight adjustments using the following guidelines. Most recipes that call for melted shortening or butter can be made using an equal amount of oil. In recipes calling for solid shortening or butter, use only seven-eighths of a cup of oil for each cup called for. In either case (melted or not), add a half teaspoon of salt to each cup of oil used. Try some of the recipes we have already adapted and you will have a better idea of what type of cake tastes best when made with oil.

Homemade pies can be excellent desserts for low-fat diets because a very flaky crust can be made with oil and the filling can be made with no saturated fat at all. You must remember that all packaged pie crust mixes contain shortening and therefore should not be used. That really isn't a problem because our crust recipes are easy to prepare— one is actually mixed right in the pie plate!

If you are in the habit of dotting your pies with butter, try sprinkling a few drops of oil as a substitute. There are many canned and packaged pie fillings available, most of which are acceptable, but check the label for the odd brand with undesirable ingredients.

Helpful Hints

Some of the recipes call for sour milk. To make sour milk, add 1½ tablespoons of lemon juice or 1⅓ tablespoons of vinegar to each cup of lukewarm skim milk and allow to stand for a few minutes before using.

We have used all-purpose flour in all of our recipes rather than self-rising flour. This gives better control over the results since the amount of baking powder or baking soda varies from recipe to recipe and can thus be measured more accurately.

When a baking pan has to be greased and you aren't using one made of Teflon, use a small amount of oil in place of butter or shortening. The new vegetable spray-on coatings provide an efficient, simple and safe way of doing the same thing.

When baking deep-dish cakes, such as our blueberry cake, cover the bottom and sides of the pan with a continuous piece of aluminum foil before adding the batter. After the cake has been baked and cooled, simply lift it out and place it on a platter. This will prevent the soft cake from disintegrating as you remove it from the pan.

One of the most important things to remember when baking our cakes, or any cake for that matter, is not to overbake. Overbaking tends to toughen and dry out a cake, and oil-based cakes are more susceptible to this than butter-based cakes, so it pays to be a little more careful. Oven temperatures vary a great deal, perhaps as much as twenty-five to forty degrees, so continually test your cakes for doneness with a toothpick near the end of the baking time. When the toothpick, inserted in the center of the cake, comes out clean and relatively dry, the cake is done.

CAKES AND BREADS
BOSTON CREAM PIE

Cake

Beat until thick and lemon-colored:

2 eggs

Add, beating constantly at medium speed, for about 3 minutes:

1 cup sugar

Then add, and stir until blended:

1 teaspoon vanilla
1 cup sifted all-purpose flour
1 teaspoon baking powder
¼ teaspoon salt

Combine and add to the flour mixture:

½ cup hot skim milk
2 tablespoons oil

Blend well. Pour batter into 2 greased and floured 8-inch round cake pans. Bake in 350° oven for 25 minutes. Cool for about 15 minutes before removing layers.

Cream Custard Filling

In saucepan combine:

⅓ cup sugar
2 tablespoons flour
1 tablespoon cornstarch
¼ teaspoon salt

Gradually stir in: **1½ cups skim milk**

Cook over moderate heat stirring constantly until mixture boils and thickens—2-3 minutes longer. Then beat slightly:

1 egg

Stir a little of the hot mixture into the egg, then return it to the pan continuing to cook and stir until mixture comes to a boil.

Add: 1 teaspoon vanilla

Cool, then beat until smooth. Spread over one layer and top with the second layer.

Chocolate Glaze

Combine: 1 cup confectioners' sugar
                     2 tablespoons unsweetened cocoa
                     3 tablespoons oil
                     ¼ teaspoon almond extract

Stir in enough boiling water (about 2 tablespoons) to make it of drizzling consistency. Spoon over cake.

BASIC CHIFFON CAKE AND VARIATIONS

Beat in a large bowl until very stiff and glossy:

                     ½ cup egg whites
                     ¼ teaspoon cream of tartar

Into a small bowl   1 cup sifted all-purpose flour
sift: ¾ cup sugar
                     1½ teaspoons baking powder
                     ½ teaspoon salt

Make a well in the flour mixture and add:
                     ¼ cup oil
                     2 egg yolks
                     ⅓ cup cold water
                     1 teaspoon vanilla

Mix with spoon just until smooth. Then fold the egg white mixture into the cake batter gently, but thoroughly. Pour into an unoiled 8-inch tube cake pan or an 8-inch square pan. Bake in 350° oven 30-40 minutes or until top springs back when lightly touched. Immediately turn upside down to hang, resting four corners on saucers. Let hang free of table until cold. Loosen sides of pan with knife and rap sharply on bottom to remove.

PARTY-SIZED CHIFFON CAKE

Double all ingredients for Basic Chiffon Cake and follow the same method. Bake in an unoiled 10-inch tube pan 4 inches deep in 325° oven for 55 minutes; then increase the heat to 350° and continue to bake 15 minutes longer or until top springs back when lightly touched.

BANANA NUT CHIFFON

Prepare the Basic Chiffon Cake recipe, adding:

¼ cup chopped nuts
½ cup mashed ripe bananas

to the dry ingredients. Bake 30-40 minutes.

MARBLE CHIFFON CAKE

Blend together with fingers, then set aside for filling:

2 tablespoons unsweetened cocoa
3 tablespoons brown sugar
1 teaspoon almond extract

Make the Basic Chiffon Cake. Sprinkle the chocolate filling in layers as you pour the batter into the pan. Bake as directed.

ORANGE CHIFFON CAKE

In the Basic Chiffon Cake recipe, substitute:

orange juice for the water

and add: **1 teaspoon grated orange rind**

Bake 30-40 minutes. Frost with a lemon glaze.

LAYER CAKE

Prepare two round 8- or 9-inch layer pans or one 9 x 13 inch pan by lightly oiling and dusting with flour.

Beat until frothy: **2 egg whites**

Gradually beat in and continue beating until very stiff and shiny:

½ cup sugar

Into another bowl sift:

1 cup sugar
2 cups sifted all-purpose flour
3 teaspoons baking powder
1 teaspoon salt

Add and beat for 1 minute:

⅓ cup oil
½ cup skim milk
1½ teaspoons vanilla

Add and beat 1 minute longer:

½ cup skim milk (another)
2 egg yolks

Gently fold in the egg white mixture. Pour into prepared pans and bake in a 350° oven 30-40 minutes for layers, 40-45 minutes for 9 x 13 inch pan.

CUPCAKES

Cupcakes may be baked in muffin pans or papers. For a birthday party make individual cupcakes and write the guest's name in icing and you have a novel place card. Makes 24.

MAGIC UPSIDE-DOWN CAKE

Mix together and set aside:	**1 tablespoon unsweetened cocoa** **⅓ cup brown sugar** **⅓ cup white sugar**
Combine in a large bowl:	**¾ cup sugar** **⅞ cup sifted all-purpose flour** **2 teaspoons baking powder** **3 tablespoons unsweetened cocoa** **¼ teaspoon salt** **¼ cup oil** **½ cup skim milk** **1 teaspoon vanilla**

Pour into a lightly oiled 8 x 8 inch pan. Over this, sprinkle the dry unsweetened cocoa and sugar mixture. Then over this pour:

¾ cup cold coffee

Bake in 350° oven for 35 minutes. Loosen around edges, then turn out on serving plate immediately, taking care not to burn yourself. This cake is "self-icing," because during the baking process, the cake rises and a fudgy sauce sinks. When turned out, this sauce becomes the icing.

BEST EVER CHOCOLATE CAKE

Put all the ingredients in a bowl and mix until smooth:	**¾ cup oil** **1½ cups sugar** **¾ cups skim milk** **6 tablespoons unsweetened cocoa** **1 cup sifted all-purpose flour** **3 teaspoons baking powder** **¼ teaspoon salt** **3 eggs** **1½ teaspoons vanilla** **1½ teaspoons cinnamon**

Pour into a lightly oiled 9 x 13 inch pan and bake in a 350° oven for 30 minutes. Ice with Seven-Minute Icing. This is the favorite birthday cake in our house.

SEVEN SISTERS YEAST CAKE

Dough—Must be refrigerated overnight.

Dissolve and set aside:	**1 package yeast**
in:	**¼ cup water**
	1 teaspoon sugar
Heat:	**½ cup skim milk**
	½ teaspoon salt
	½ cup sugar
Remove from heat and add:	**¾ cup oil**
	2 eggs
	½ cup "sour cream" (see recipe) or natural-flavored skim milk yogurt
	3 cups sifted all-purpose flour
	the yeast mixture

Mix dough well. Cover and leave in refrigerator overnight.

Fruit Filling—Cover with water for a few hours or overnight.

	1 cup pitted prunes cut in pieces
	2 tablespoons mixed fruit peel
	½ cup dried apricots cut in pieces
When ready to proceed, heat until bubbly:	**1 cup brown sugar**
	4 tablespoons oil
	3 tablespoons juice from the soaked fruit
	1 teaspoon cinnamon

Pour a little of this syrup in the bottom of an oiled, 2-quart, fluted tube pan.

To the remaining syrup add:	**drained prune mixture**
	½ cup raisins
	¼ cup cut-up, toasted almonds

Roll dough on a well-floured board into a rectangle about half an inch thick. Spread fruit on dough; roll as for jelly roll. Cut in 7 pieces and place side by side in a pan, alternating cut side up. Let rise in a warm place for 1-2 hours or until doubled in bulk. Bake in a 350° oven for 1-1¼ hours until well baked. Allow to cool for about 30 minutes and then invert on your prettiest cake platter.

"SOUR CREAM" COFFEE CAKE

Beat:	**¼ cup oil**
	1 cup sugar
	3 eggs (less 1 yolk)

In another bowl, sift:	1¾ cups sifted all-purpose flour ½ teaspoon baking soda 2 teaspoons baking powder ½ teaspoon salt

Add the sifted dry ingredients to the oil mixture, alternating with:

1 cup "sour cream" (see recipe) or natural-flavored skim milk yogurt

Pour half the dough into a lightly oiled, 9-inch square pan and sprinkle dough with a mixture made from:

½ cup brown sugar
½ cup raisins
a few broken walnut halves
1 teaspoon cinnamon

Cover with remaining dough. Then blend the following together with your fingers:

2 tablespoons sugar
½ teaspoon cinnamon
1 tablespoon flour
1 teaspoon oil

and sprinkle it over the cake. Bake in 350° oven for 30-45 minutes.

GRAHAM MOCHA LAYER CAKE OR SQUARES

Beat:	¾ cup oil 1 cup sugar 3 eggs (less 1 yolk)
Add:	2 cups graham cracker crumbs 3½ teaspoons baking powder 3 tablespoons sifted all-purpose flour ¼ teaspoon salt 1 cup skim milk 1 teaspoon vanilla

Mix at low speed until well blended. This will be a very loose batter. Pour cake into 2 lightly oiled 8-inch round pans, or in a 9 x 13 inch pan. Bake in a 400° oven 15-20 minutes. When cool, ice with Coffee Icing Glaze. When making a layer cake, crushed pineapple, slightly drained makes a lovely filling.

Coffee Icing Glaze

Beat together:	1 tablespoon oil 1 teaspoon instant coffee

dissolved in: **1 tablespoon cold water**
                       1 cup icing sugar
Thin with: **skim milk**

adding very little at a time until thin enough to spread easily. For a layer cake, make 1½ times this recipe.

LEMON POUND CAKE

Mix thoroughly   **¾ cup icing sugar**
and set aside: **¾ cup lemon juice**
                      rind of half a lemon, finely grated

Beat well: **½ cup oil**
                      1½ cups sugar

Add and continue beating:

                      3 eggs

Sift together   **2 cups sifted all-purpose flour**
and add: **1½ teaspoons baking powder**
                      pinch of salt

Then add: **½ teaspoon almond extract**
                      ¼ teaspoon lemon rind
                      ¾ cup skim milk

Bake in a lightly oiled bundt pan or tube pan in a 350° oven for 1 hour. While hot, pierce many times with a cake tester or toothpick and spoon lemon juice mixture over the cake until all is absorbed.

APPLESAUCE CAKE

Beat: **1 cup sugar**
                      ⅓ cup oil
                      1 egg

Add: **1 cup sweetened applesauce**

Sift together: **1¾ cups sifted all-purpose flour**
                      1 teaspoon salt
                      1 teaspoon baking soda
                      1 teaspoon cinnamon
                      pinch of allspice
                      pinch of nutmeg

Sift part of this   **1 cup raisins**
mixture over: **1 cup currants or chopped dates**

Add the rest of the flour gradually to the batter. Beat until smooth. Fold in raisins and currants. Place batter in a lightly oiled 9 x 13 inch pan. Bake in a 350° oven for 40 minutes. You can sprinkle a little confectioners' sugar over the cake when it is cool.

BLUEBERRY CAKE

Beat until smooth: ¾ cup oil
¾ cup sugar
2 eggs
2 tablespoons water
1 teaspoon vanilla
¼ teaspoon salt

Add: 1½ cups sifted all-purpose flour
2 teaspoons baking powder

Pour ¾ of batter in a lightly oiled 9 x 13 inch pan.

Mix together: 1 can blueberry pie filling (20 ounces)
2 teaspoons cornstarch, mixed with
2 teaspoons lemon juice
grated rind of ½ lemon

Spread over dough by spoonfuls.

To remaining
batter add: 2 or 3 teaspoons water to thin

Drizzle batter over blueberries. Sprinkle:

cinnamon-sugar

over the top.

Bake in 350° oven for 45-60 minutes. Cut into 3-inch squares. Cherry or any other pie filling may be substituted for the blueberry.

PINEAPPLE PECAN CAKE

Combine in bowl
and beat 1 minute: 1 cup sugar
1 teaspoon vanilla
2 eggs

Add and continue
beating until well
mixed: 2 cups sifted all-purpose flour
1 teaspoon salt
1 teaspoon baking soda
1 can crushed pineapple, undrained (14 ounces)

Pour batter into lightly oiled 9 x 13 inch pan and sprinkle with a mixture of:

½ cup firmly packed brown sugar
¾ cup chopped pecans
4 drops coconut flavoring (optional)

Bake in 350° oven 30-40 minutes. Remove cake from oven and pierce top many times with cake tester or toothpick and pour sauce slowly and evenly over the hot cake.

Sauce

Stir until sugar is dissolved and set aside:

> ¼ cup oil
> ½ cup skim milk
> ½ cup sugar
> ½ teaspoon vanilla

QUICK APPLE CAKE

Into a lightly oiled 9 x 12 inch Pyrex dish, arrange:

> **10 apples, peeled and sliced**

Sprinkle with generous amounts of:

> cinnamon
> brown sugar
> juice of half a lemon

Set aside.

Beat well:

> ¾ cup oil
> ¾ cup sugar
> 2 eggs

Sift together and add:

> 1½ cups sifted all-purpose flour
> 2 teaspoons baking powder
> ¼ teaspoon salt

Then add:

> 1 teaspoon vanilla
> 3 tablespoons water

Spread dough evenly over the apples—a flat knife dipped in water will help you do this. Sprinkle dough with a mixture of:

> 2 grated walnut halves
> 2 tablespoons sugar
> 1 teaspoon cinnamon

Bake in a 350° oven for 45 minutes.

CHERRY CUSTARD CAKE

Beat together until light and fluffy:

> 2 eggs
> ½ cup sugar
> ½ cup oil
> ⅛ teaspoon salt

Then add:

> 2½ cups sifted all-purpose flour
> 1 teaspoon vanilla
> 2 teaspoons baking powder

Pat ⅔ of dough into a spring form covering bottom and about 2½ inches up the sides.

Cook as directed on package using skim milk:

1 package vanilla pudding (3 ounces)

Pour pudding over dough.

Drain, reserving juice, and then arrange over custard:

1 can red pitted cherries (19 ounces)

Roll balance of dough into long strips and make a lattice design over cherries.

Combine: **½ cup sugar**
4 teaspoons cornstarch
1 teaspoon almond extract

Add: **reserved cherry juice (there should be about ¾ cup)**

Cook slowly until clear and thickened, stirring constantly, then pour over cake. Bake in 350° oven 45-60 minutes or until well baked.

CHOCOLATE JELLY ROLL

Beat in large bowl until thick and lemon colored (about 5 minutes at high speed):

3 eggs

Gradually beat in: **1 cup sugar**

Blend in: **⅓ cup water**
1 teaspoon vanilla

Sift together, then beat in just until batter is smooth:

1 cup less 2 tablespoons all-purpose flour
1 teaspoon baking powder
¼ teaspoon salt
¼ cup unsweetened cocoa

Pour into jelly roll pan that has been oiled and lined with oiled waxed paper. Bake 12-15 minutes in moderate 350° oven. Do not overbake. Sprinkle top of cake with a little sifted cocoa. Loosen edges and turn out on clean towel. Peel off paper and trim off crisp edges if necessary. Roll in towel from narrow end while hot. Cool. Unroll when cool and fill with Orange Filling. Reroll cake and sprinkle top with sifted confectioners' sugar.

SPONGE CAKE JELLY ROLL AND VARIATIONS

Beat with electric mixer for about 5 minutes:

4 eggs (less one yolk)

Gradually add: **1 cup sugar**

Sift together and then fold into egg mixture:

1 cup less 2 tablespoons sifted all-purpose flour
1 teaspoon baking powder
¼ teaspoon salt

Spread the dough in a 15 x 10 inch jelly roll pan that has been oiled and lined with oiled waxed paper. Bake in 400° oven for 10-15 minutes. While hot, invert the cake onto a tea towel that has been sprinkled with:

1 tablespoon confectioners' sugar

Remove the paper, roll the cake in the towel and cool. When cool, unroll, spread the cake with:

1 cup jelly or a tart jam

and reroll. Before serving, sprinkle with powdered sugar.

LEMON-STRAWBERRY ROLL

Fill the above roll with:

Lemon Filling

to which has been added:

½ cup fresh strawberries

Refrigerate until serving time and before serving garnish with:

confectioners' sugar
fresh berries

MOCHA NUT ROLL

To the sponge cake jelly roll dough, add:

⅓ cup chopped nuts (walnuts or pecans)

Bake as above. Fill with Mocha Cream Filling. Refrigerate until serving time and sprinkle with:

confectioners' sugar

These are a few of our favorite variations. You can use any number of combinations that will be equally delicious.

CRUMB SPICE CAKE

Combine until
crumbly:
⅔ cup oil
2½ cups sifted all-purpose flour
2 cups dark brown sugar

Reserve one cup of these crumbs. To the remainder add:

½ teaspoon baking soda
½ teaspoon salt
¼ teaspoon nutmeg

½ teaspoon cinnamon
2 teaspoons baking powder

Then add and
mix thoroughly:
1 cup sour milk
2 eggs

Spread in lightly oiled 9 x 13 inch pan.

To the reserved
crumbs add:
¾ teaspoon cinnamon
¼ cup blanched, shredded almonds

Sprinkle these crumbs over dough, and bake in 350° oven 30 minutes.

SPICED PRUNE CAKE

Beat until light:
1 cup sugar
½ cup oil

Add, one at a time:
2 eggs

Beat in:
1 cup prunes, cooked and mashed

Sift together:
1⅓ cups sifted all-purpose flour
1½ teaspoons baking soda
1 teaspoon cinnamon
¾ teaspoon cloves
½ teaspoon salt

Add sifted ingredients in three parts alternately with:

½ cup sour milk

Beat after each addition until smooth. Pour into a lightly oiled 9 x 13 inch pan. Bake in 350° oven 20-30 minutes. Ice with Seven-Minute Icing.

DARK FRUIT CAKE

Boil together for
5 minutes:
1½ cups raisins
¼ cup oil
¾ cup sugar
½ teaspoon cinnamon
¼ teaspoon nutmeg
¼ teaspoon allspice
grated rind of 1 small orange
½ cup mixed peels, fruits, and cherries
1 cup cold water

When cool, pour
into mixing bowl
and add:
1 cup sifted all-purpose flour
½ teaspoon baking soda
½ teaspoon unsweetened cocoa
¼ cup broken walnuts
½ teaspoon salt

Pour into lightly oiled 8 x 8 inch pan. Bake in 350° oven for about 1 hour. This recipe contains no eggs.

CHRISTMAS FRUITCAKE

This is a delicious, moist fruitcake. It should be made weeks in advance to allow it to mellow and ripen.

Combine and beat for two minutes:	**1 cup oil** **1½ cups brown sugar** **4 eggs**
Sift:	**2 cups sifted all-purpose flour** **1 teaspoon baking powder** **2 teaspoons salt** **2 teaspoons cinnamon** **2 teaspoons allspice** **1 teaspoon cloves**

Stir the dry ingredients into the oil mixture alternately with:

1 cup orange juice

Mix together:	**1 cup sifted all-purpose flour** **1 cup chopped dates** **1 cup raisins** **1 cup candied cherries (the whole ones look nice)** **1 cup chopped, candied pineapple** **1 cup thinly sliced citron** **3 cups chopped walnuts**

Pour the batter over the fruit, mixing thoroughly. Pour into two loaf pans (approximately 8 x 4 x 2 inches), that have been lightly oiled and lined with oiled brown paper. Place a pan of water on the lower oven rack. Bake the cakes for 2½-3 hours in a 275° oven. After they have baked, let them stand for about 20 minutes before removing them from the pans. Cool them thoroughly on racks without removing the paper. When cool, remove the paper, wrap in aluminum foil, and store to ripen. If desired, the cakes can be wrapped in cloth dampened in brandy. The cloth must be redampened every week. Chill the cake an hour or two before slicing.

RAISIN-NUT LOAF

Combine in a small bowl:	**1 cup boiling water** **2 cups raisins** **10 finely cut dried apricots (optional)**
Add: and allow to cool.	**1 tablespoon oil**
Beat in a large bowl:	**2 eggs** **⅔ cup sugar** **1 teaspoon vanilla**
Add and mix well:	**2 cups sifted all-purpose flour** **1 rounded teaspoon baking soda** **⅛ teaspoon salt**

Then add:	cooled raisin mixture
	½ cup walnuts, chopped

Mix thoroughly and pour into lightly oiled loaf pan. Bake in 350° oven for about 1 hour. If desired, slice and store in plastic bag in freezer. Slices may then be removed individually.

CRANBERRY-ORANGE BREAD

Sift together:	2 cups sifted all-purpose flour
	1½ teaspoons baking powder
	½ teaspoon baking soda
	½ teaspoon salt
	1 cup sugar
Add, mixing thoroughly:	2 tablespoons oil
	grated rind and juice of one orange plus orange juice to make ¾ cup
	1 egg, beaten
Fold in:	1 cup raw cranberries cut in half

Pour into greased 9 x 5 x 3 inch loaf pan. Bake in 350° oven for about 1 hour, until toothpick stuck into center comes out clean.

CHERRY-NUT LOAF

Beat:	2 eggs
	¼ cup maraschino cherry juice
	¾ cup skim milk
	3 tablespoons oil
	¼ teaspoon almond extract
Sift:	2 cups sifted all-purpose flour
	1 cup sugar
	3 teaspoons baking powder
	½ teaspoon salt

Stir the liquid mixture into the dry mixture and beat until smooth, about 30 seconds.

Then stir in:	1 cup maraschino cherries, cut in half
	½ cup chopped walnuts

Spoon into a greased 9 x 5 x 3 inch loaf pan. Bake in 350° oven for about 1 hour (or until a toothpick inserted in the center comes out clean).

BANANA-NUT LOAF

Beat:	½ cup oil
	1 cup sugar
Add:	2 beaten eggs
	1 cup mashed bananas (about 3)

Beat well.

Sift together: **2 cups sifted all-purpose flour**
1 teaspoon baking soda
½ teaspoon baking powder
½ teaspoon salt

and add to the oil mixture.

Then add: **3 tablespoons skim milk**
½ teaspoon vanilla

Beat well and stir in:

½ cup chopped walnuts

Bake in a lightly oiled 9 x 5 x 3 inch loaf pan in a 350° oven about 1 hour. Cool well and store in an airtight container.

DATE LOAF

This is by far the best date loaf we have ever tasted. See what your family and friends think.

In a large bowl sprinkle:

½ teaspoon baking soda

over: **½ pound pitted, finely chopped dates**

Then add: **1 cup boiling water**
½ cup oil

In another bowl sift the following together and then stir into date mixture:

1 cup sugar
1½ cups sifted all-purpose flour
2 teaspoons baking powder
½ teaspoon salt

Add and mix thoroughly: **½ cup chopped walnuts**
½ cup cut mixed peel, finely chopped
½ teaspoon vanilla
2 eggs, well beaten
grated rind of 1 orange

Pour into an oiled 9 x 5 x 3 inch loaf pan. Bake in a 350° oven for 1 hour or until cake tester comes out clean. Remove from the oven.

Combine: **3 tablespoons sugar**
¼ cup orange juice

Pour over hot cake. Cool cake in pan. This cake freezes very well if your family doesn't finish it first.

APRICOT-NUT BREAD

Cover and soak in boiling water for 15 minutes:

¾ cup dried apricots, cut into pieces

Drain the apricots, reserving liquid, adding enough:

orange juice

to make 1 cup of liquid.

Sift:
- **2 cups sifted all-purpose flour**
- **2 teaspoons baking powder**
- **¼ teaspoon baking soda**
- **½ teaspoon salt**
- **1 cup sugar**

Add:
- **1 cup apricot orange liquid (reserved above)**
- **1 teaspoon grated orange rind**
- **drained apricots**
- **1 egg**
- **2 tablespoons oil**

Beat gently until blended.

Fold in: **½ cup chopped nuts**

Bake in a lightly oiled 9 x 5 x 3 inch loaf pan in a 350° oven for about 1 hour.

JOHNNY CAKE

Preheat oven to 425°. Grease a 9 x 5 x 3 inch loaf pan or 12 muffin tins with:

2 tablespoons oil

and place in oven to heat for 3 minutes before adding the batter.

Combine:
- **1 cup sifted all-purpose flour**
- **1 cup yellow cornmeal**
- **½ teaspoon salt**
- **2 teaspoons baking powder**
- **¼ cup sugar**

Combine and add:
- **¾ cup skim milk**
- **1 egg**
- **½ cup oil**

Stir only until flour is dampened. Pour batter into hot loaf pan or muffin tins. Bake in 425° oven for 30-40 minutes.

For Corn Toasties bake as above in 9 x 13 pan for 15-20 minutes. Cut into squares.

GINGERBREAD

Beat:	½ cup sugar ½ cup oil 2 well-beaten eggs
Add:	1 cup molasses 2 teaspoons baking soda dissolved in 1 cup boiling water
Then add:	2½ cups sifted all-purpose flour ½ teaspoon salt 1 teaspoon ginger ½ teaspoon cinnamon ¼ teaspoon cloves

Mix until all lumps are gone. This is a soft batter. Pour into a lightly oiled 9 x 13 inch pan and bake in a 350° oven for about 30 minutes. Cut into squares.

BANANA BRAN MUFFINS

Soak and set aside:	1 cup whole bran in 1 cup buttermilk or sour milk
Beat:	2 tablespoons oil ¼ cup sugar 1 egg ¾ cup mashed bananas (about 2 large) ¼ cup raisins
Sift and add alternately with bran mixture:	1½ cups sifted all-purpose flour ½ teaspoon baking soda 1 teaspoon baking powder 1 teaspoon cinnamon ½ teaspoon salt

Stir only until blended. Fill muffin tins only ¾ full. Bake in 400° oven 15-20 minutes.

BREAKFAST MUFFINS AND VARIATIONS

Sift:	2 cups sifted all-purpose flour ¼ cup sugar 3 teaspoons baking powder 1 teaspoon salt
Make a well and add:	1 egg, well beaten 1 cup skim milk ¼ cup oil

Stir only to dampen flour. Batter should be lumpy. Fill lightly oiled muffin cups or muffin papers only ⅔ full. Bake at 400° for 25 minutes. Makes 12 muffins.

Variations

Blueberry Muffins—Add ½ cup fresh, or drained canned or frozen blueberries to the above batter.

Cherry Nut Muffins—Add ½ cup quartered maraschino cherries, patted dry, ¼ cup chopped nuts, and ¼ teaspoon almond extract to the above batter.

Jam Muffins—Fill muffin cups ⅓ full, and add 1 teaspoon of any jam or marmalade. Cover with batter to fill cups ⅔ full.

Pineapple Muffins—Add ½ cup well-drained crushed pineapple to the above batter.

Banana Muffins—Add ½ cup mashed bananas to the batter.

These are some of the variations that we use. No doubt your family will have their own favorites. These muffins freeze well and may be warmed up in the oven quickly. It's a good idea to have lots on hand for snacks, breakfasts, lunch treats, or to put in a lunchbox.

APPLE MUFFINS

Combine:	**1 cup sugar**
	⅔ cup oil
	2 eggs
Add:	**1 cup skim milk**
	¼ teaspoon almond extract
Then add and beat until smooth:	**2 cups sifted all-purpose flour**
	2 teaspoons baking powder
	¼ teaspoon salt
	½ teaspoon cinnamon
Add, mixing well:	**1 cup apples, peeled and diced**

Fill muffin cups ⅔ full. Bake in 350° oven 25-30 minutes.

CINNAMON-NUT ROLLS

Combine and sprinkle over bottom of 18 lightly oiled muffin tins and set aside:

	½ cup brown sugar
	¼ cup chopped nuts
	¼ cup oil
In a large bowl, sift:	**3 cups sifted all-purpose flour**
	¼ teaspoon salt

3½ teaspoons baking powder
½ cup sugar

Combine and add
to the dry   **1 cup skim milk**
ingredients: **½ cup oil**

Mix well. Place dough on a lightly floured board, knead lightly about ten times. Roll into a rectangular shape about ¼-inch thick. Spread generously with a mixture of:

2 tablespoons oil
½ cup brown sugar
1 teaspoon cinnamon

Roll dough as for jelly roll. Cut into 1-inch slices. Place slices cut side down in prepared pans. Bake in 350° oven for 25-30 minutes in top third of oven. These may be prepared up to the point of baking and refrigerated overnight. Next morning pop them into the oven and have hot rolls for breakfast!

BASIC BAKING POWDER BISCUIT MIX

Combine until   **8 cups flour**
the texture of   **1 tablespoon salt**
fine meal: **¼ cup baking powder**
                       1 cup skim milk powder
                       1 cup oil

Store in covered jar in refrigerator. It will keep for weeks.

Biscuits:

Measure: **2 cups lightly packed mix**

Add: **⅓ cup skim milk**
                  2 teaspoons chives (optional)

Stir quickly, and turn out on a lightly floured board. Knead gently 15 or 20 times. Roll out ¼ to ½-inch thick. Cut rounds with biscuit cutter, or cut squares with a lightly floured knife. Place biscuits an inch apart, if you like them crusty, close together if you don't. Bake 10-12 minutes in 425° oven.

For a breakfast roll, pat dough ¼-inch thick and sprinkle generously with:

brown sugar
oil
cinnamon
seedless raisins

Roll as for jelly roll, slice ¾-inch thick, place cut side down, and bake as above.

BAKING POWDER BISCUITS WITH VARIATIONS

Basic Dough

Sift together and make a well:	**2 cups sifted all-purpose flour** **3 teaspoons baking powder** **1 teaspoon salt**

Pour together into a cup, but do not stir:	**⅓ cup oil** **⅔ cup skim milk**

Pour liquids into the well all at once and stir with a fork until mixture cleans side of bowl. On a floured board knead dough about 10 times. Roll out ¼- or ½-inch thick. Cut with a floured biscuit cutter. Place on an ungreased cookie sheet. Bake in 450° oven for 10-12 minutes. For soft biscuits, place biscuits close together with sides touching. For crusty biscuits, place well apart.

Drop Biscuits

Prepare dough as above and drop unkneaded dough from spoon onto ungreased cookie sheet. Bake as above.

Cinnamon Raisin Biscuits

Add to the dry ingredients:	**¼ teaspoon cinnamon** **¼ teaspoon nutmeg** **⅓ cup currants or raisins**

Bake as above.

Chive Biscuits

Add to the dry ingredients:

2 tablespons chopped chives

Bake as above.

TOAST POINTS

Lightly brush:	**triangles of bread**
with:	**oil**
Sprinkle with any of the following:	**garlic salt** **celery salt** **salad herbs**

Broil until golden. Serve hot.

GARLIC BREAD

| Combine in a
small jar: | ⅓ cup oil
¼ teaspoon salt
2 cloves garlic, sliced |

Allow to stand about 30 minutes and then remove the garlic.

| Slice: | 1 loaf French bread |

into 2-inch slices, cutting to within one-quarter inch of the bottom crust. Pull the slices slightly apart and brush the cut surfaces with the oil. Wrap the loaf in a piece of aluminum foil. Bake in 350° oven for about 20 minutes, or until the loaf is heated through.

ONION BREAD

Slice diagonally in thick slices to within one-quarter inch of the bottom crust:

French or Italian bread

Lightly brush both sides of each slice with:

oil

and sprinkle with: **dry onion soup mix**

Wrap in aluminum foil. Place on a baking sheet in a hot oven, 350° for about 15 minutes. Serve hot with a tossed salad, breaking off one slice at a time.

COOKIES AND SQUARES

"CHOCOLATE" CHIP COOKIES

Chips

| In a small bowl,
blend together
with a spoon: | ¼ cup unsweetened cocoa
¼ cup brown sugar
4 teaspoons oil
1 teaspoon vanilla |

The mixture should be very thick, but not crumbly. If it is too moist, add ½ teaspoon cocoa and brown sugar, and if too dry, add more oil drop by drop. Flatten the mixture on a breadboard about ⅛-inch thick and cut into chip-sized squares. Allow to dry for a few hours or overnight and store in a covered jar. Makes about ½ cup of chips.

Cookies

| Beat: | 1 egg
½ cup oil
1 teaspoon vanilla |

Add and continue beating:	¼ cup brown sugar ½ cup granulated sugar
Then add:	1 cup sifted all-purpose flour ½ teaspoon baking soda ½ teaspoon salt
Gently fold in:	½ cup "chocolate" chips

Drop by the spoonful 2 inches apart on a lightly oiled cookie sheet. Bake in 375° oven for about 8 minutes.

SUGAR COOKIES

| In a mixing bowl, combine: | ¾ cup oil
1 cup sugar |

Add one at a time beating well after each addition:

2 eggs
1 teaspoon vanilla

| Sift together and add all at once: | 2½ cups sifted all-purpose flour
1½ teaspoons baking powder
½ teaspoon salt |

Blend well. Shape dough into balls, about 1 inch in diameter. Dip the tops of the balls in any of the following:

granulated sugar
colored sugar
candy sprinkles

Place balls of dough, sugar side up, 3 inches apart on an ungreased cookie sheet. Press cookies with fork to flatten dough. Bake in a 375° oven 10-12 minutes. Remove immediately from cookie sheet. Makes about 5 dozen cookies.

This dough can also be rolled and cut with cookie cutters, and then baked as above. These are favorites with the children in our house because they love to cut and decorate the cookies themselves.

GINGER-HONEY SNAPS

Beat in a large bowl:	⅔ cup oil 1 cup sugar 1 egg
Stir in:	¼ cup honey
Sift together and then add:	2 cups sifted all-purpose flour 2 teaspoons baking soda 1 teaspoon ground ginger (more if desired) ⅛ teaspoon salt

Shape the dough into rolls the diameter of a quarter and then slice ½-inch thick. Dip each slice in:

granulated sugar

Place cookies 1 inch apart on ungreased cookie sheet. Bake 12-15 minutes in 350° oven. Let stand about 1 minute before removing from cookie sheet.

CHOCOLATE CRINKLE COOKIES

Beat together:
- ½ cup oil
- 2 eggs
- 1 cup sugar
- 1 teaspoon vanilla
- 1 teaspoon almond extract

Sift together and add blending well:
- ¼ teaspoon salt
- 1 cup sifted all-purpose flour
- 1 teaspoon baking powder
- 4 tablespoons unsweetened cocoa

Refrigerate dough overnight. Drop small balls of dough into:

confectioners' sugar

Place them on a cookie sheet at least 2 inches apart. Bake in 400° oven 8-10 minutes. Do not overbake. This is a lovely rainy day project for the children to help with. Makes about 5 dozen cookies.

SCHNECKEN AND ALMOND TWISTS

From this recipe you can make two different and delicious kinds of cookies.

Beat together:
- 1 cup oil
- 2 eggs
- 3 tablespoons sugar
- ½ teaspoon salt

Add:
- 2¼ cups sifted all-purpose flour

Add, blending well:
- 1 package of yeast (that has been dissolved by placing a teaspoon sugar in ½ cup warm water, adding the yeast, and allowing it to sit 10 minutes)

Cover the dough and refrigerate overnight. The next day, remove 1 tablespoon dough at a time and roll into a circle on a lightly floured board, as thinly as possible. Cut the circles into eighths. Place small amount of "filling" on the outer edge of each eighth and roll up twisting slightly to form a crescent. Bake in 350° oven until golden, about 8-10 minutes.

Fillings

Use one or more, or your own ideas.

Cottage cheese
Cinnamon, sugar and raisins
Jam and chopped nuts
Almond filling

ALMOND TWISTS

Almond Filling

Combine:
1 egg, slightly beaten
¾ cup sugar
½ cup bread crumbs
½ cup blanched grated or ground almonds
1½ teaspoons almond extract
2 tablespoons water

Using some of the dough from Schnecken, roll 3 pieces of dough as thin as possible into 3 x 9 inch rectangles for layers. Spread almond filling between each layer. Slice ¼-inch wide. Twist and place on cookie sheet. Bake in 350° oven until golden.

Both of these freeze very well and are worth the effort involved.

CHINESE ALMOND COOKIES

Combine:
1 cup oil
1 cup sugar
1 egg
3 cups sifted all-purpose flour
1½ teaspoons baking soda
3 TABLESPOONS almond extract
1 tablespoon corn syrup, honey or molasses

Roll into small balls and place on cookie sheet. Flatten slightly with a fork.

Press:
1 blanched almond

into each cookie. Bake in 375° oven for about 10 minutes or until golden.

CINNAMON PRETZELS

Combine and
blend well:
1 cup sugar
¾ cup oil
3 eggs, less 1 yolk

Sift together and
stir into the above:
3½ cups sifted all-purpose flour
2 teaspoons baking powder

Using floured hands, roll pieces of dough into long pencil-thick rolls, about 12 inches long. Dip into a mixture of:

> ½ cup sugar
> 1 teaspoon cinnamon

Twist into pretzel shapes. Place on a lightly oiled baking sheet, and bake in a 375° oven for 10-12 minutes. These cookies can be shaped into wreaths and decorated with candied cherries for Christmas.

POPPY SEED COOKIES

Beat:	2 eggs
Add:	⅔ cup sugar
	½ cup oil
	grated rind of an orange
	2 tablespoons orange juice
Sift together and add:	3 cups sifted all-purpose flour
	1½ teaspoons baking powder
	½ teaspoon salt
Blend well and then add:	¼ cup poppy seeds

Roll out on a floured board as thinly as possible, using as little flour as possible to handle dough. Cut into desired shapes and bake in a 350° oven for about 10 minutes or until golden.

CINNAMON RAISIN WIND-UPS

Beat well:	½ cup oil
	½ cup sugar
	2 eggs, less one yolk
	grated rind and juice of 1 orange
Sift together and then add:	2½ cups sifted all-purpose flour
	2 teaspoons baking powder
	¼ teaspoon salt

Roll ¼ of the dough at a time about ¼-inch thick on a floured board, using as little flour as possible.

Sprinkle generously with:	chopped walnuts
	cinnamon
	brown sugar
	raisins

Roll tightly as for a jelly roll. Cut ½-inch slices. Place slices cut side down on an ungreased cookie sheet. Pinch ends together slightly. Bake in 350° oven until golden, about 10-15 minutes. These freeze beautifully.

MANDEL OR ALMOND BREAD

Beat well until thick and lemon colored:

2 eggs

Add gradually, beating constantly:

⅔ cup sugar

Next add:
⅓ cup oil
½ teaspoon almond extract
1 teaspoon vanilla

Sift together
and stir in:
2 cups sifted all-purpose flour
2 teaspoons baking powder
⅛ teaspoon salt
¾ teaspoon cinnamon

Then add:
2 tablespoons orange juice
grated rind of an orange
1 cup chopped almonds

Blend well—dough will be sticky. Oil hands well and form dough into 4 loaves about 2 inches in width. Place at least 3 inches apart on a lightly oiled cookie sheet. Bake in 350° oven for 25 minutes until a light golden brown. Remove hot loaves to cutting board. While still hot cut into ½-inch slices. Reduce heat to 250°. Place slices flat side down on cookie sheets and return to oven for 10-15 minutes or until lightly toasted. Store in a tightly covered container.

OATMEAL DROP COOKIES

Beat until fluffy:
½ cup oil
1 cup brown sugar
2 eggs

Stir in:
¼ cup skim milk (skim milk yogurt or buttermilk
may be substituted)

Sift together
and add:
½ teaspoon baking soda
½ teaspoon cinnamon
¼ teaspoon salt
1 cup sifted all-purpose flour

Stir in:
1½ cups quick cooking oats

Now add two cups
of any of the
following:
raisins
nuts
mixed peel
candied cherries
snipped dates

Drop from rounded teaspoon 2 inches apart on a lightly oiled cookie sheet. Top each cookie with a:

halved candied cherry

Bake in a 350° oven for 10 to 12 minutes. Remove from cookie sheet and cool.

FLORENTINES

Stir together:	**6 tablespoons skim milk** **¼ cup oil** **3 tablespoons sugar**
Then add:	**⅓ cup slivered almonds** **⅔ cup diced candied orange peel** **¼ cup sifted all-purpose flour** **½ teaspoon baking powder** **pinch of salt**

Combine well. Oil a cookie sheet and then flour lightly. Drop dough by small spoonfuls onto the cookie sheet, well apart and spread in thin rounds. Bake in 350° oven 10-12 minutes, until golden brown. They burn easily, so watch them. Allow to cool on cookie sheet a minute or two before removing to cake rack. When cookies have cooled, spread the bottom side of the cookie with Chocolate Yogurt Icing. Place bottom side up to dry

PRUNE SURPRISES

Prepare and set aside:	**1 cup chopped raw prunes** **1 tablespoon marmalade or corn syrup to make up to the consistency of thick jam**
Beat until light and fluffy:	**1 egg** **½ cup oil** **⅔ cup brown sugar** **¼ cup molasses**
Add gradually:	**2 cups sifted all-purpose flour** **1 teaspoon baking soda** **½ teaspoon cinnamon** **½ teaspoon salt**

Chill 1-2 hours. Flatten 1 teaspoon of dough for each cookie. Place ½ teaspoon prune mixture in center, shaping dough around it. Moisten top of cookie with water and dip in granulated sugar. Place sugar side up on an ungreased cookie sheet. Bake in 350° oven for 12-15 minutes.

MARGUERITES

Make very small cupcakes (see recipe in this chapter). With a small paring knife scoop out a cone-shaped piece from center. Place 1 teaspoon Tart Lemon Filling in hole and replace top. Sprinkle with confectioners' sugar.

ORIENTAL CRUNCH

Blend together:
    ¾ cup oil
    2 tablespoons instant coffee granules *
    ½ teaspoon salt
    ½ teaspoon almond extract
    1 teaspoon vanilla
    1 cup granulated sugar
    2 cups sifted all-purpose flour

Pat firmly into a 10 x 15 inch cookie sheet. Sprinkle with and press into dough:

    ½ cup coarsely chopped almonds

Score unbaked dough into 1½-inch squares. Bake 15-20 minutes in 375° oven. Recut while hot.

CINNAMON SUGAR SHORTBREADS

Combine:
    1 egg yolk
    1 tablespoon white vinegar
    ½ teaspoon vanilla
    ½ teaspoon almond extract

Add, blending well:
    ⅔ cup oil
    ⅔ cup sugar

Then add, mixing until well blended:
    2½ cups sifted all-purpose flour
    ½ teaspoon salt
    ¼ teaspoon baking soda

This is a very dry, crumbly dough. Press down on cookie sheet or jelly roll pan to thickness of about ⅛ inch. If your pan is small, use part of a second one. Roll dough with flat-sided glass or jar as thinly as possible. Score dough into desired shapes.

Beat until frothy: **1 egg white**

Brush on dough with pastry brush and sprinkle with mixture of:

    cinnamon and sugar

Bake in 400° oven 5-10 minutes until golden brown. Recut along scored lines while warm. This cookie freezes very well and is a most delicious shortbread.

SPICED ALMOND AND FRUIT CRISPS

Beat together:
    ½ cup oil
    1 cup brown sugar

---

* If coffee granules are coarse, as in freeze-dried coffee, crush fine before using.

                              1 teaspoon vanilla
                              1 egg yolk

Sift and then add: 1¾ cups sifted all-purpose flour
                              ¼ teaspoon salt
                              ¼ teaspoon baking soda

Pat dough onto cookie sheet (11 x 15 inches).

Beat until frothy: 1 egg white

Add: 2 tablespoons granulated sugar
                              ½ teaspoon cinnamon
                              ¼ teaspoon ground nutmeg
                              ⅛ teaspoon ground cloves
                              ½ cup mixed, cut-up candied fruit
                              1 cup thinly sliced almonds

Spread over dough and bake 15 minutes in 350° oven. Cut into squares while hot.

ELLEN'S BROWNIES

Beat: 4 eggs, less 1 yolk

Add gradually: 2 cups sugar

Then add: 1 cup oil
                              2 teaspoons vanilla

Add all at once,   ⅔ cup of unsweetened cocoa
blending well: 1½ cups sifted all-purpose flour
                              1 teaspoon baking powder
                              1 teaspoon salt
                              ¼ cup of walnuts (if desired)

Put in a lightly oiled 9 x 13 inch pan. Bake at 350° for 30 minutes. Do not overbake so they will be fudgy.

BROWNIES #2

A slightly less rich brownie, but also very good—try them both.

Beat: 3 eggs

Add: 1½ cups sugar
                              ¾ cup oil
                              1½ teaspoons almond extract

Then add: 1 cup plus 2 tablespoons sifted all-purpose flour
                              1 teaspoon salt
                              ¾ teaspoon baking powder
                              ½ cup unsweetened cocoa
                              ½ cup chopped walnuts

Pour into a lightly oiled 9 x 13 inch pan. Bake in 350° oven for 20 minutes. Before serving, place

1 tablespoon confectioners' sugar

in fine strainer and shake over brownies.

CHOCOLATE MERINGUE SQUARES

Base

Blend together:	**¾ cup oil** **1 cup sugar** **2 eggs, less 1 yolk**
Add, blending well:	**1¾ cups sifted all-purpose flour** **1½ teaspoons baking powder** **1 teaspoon almond extract** **⅛ teaspoon salt**

Spread into a lightly oiled 9 x 13 inch pan and set aside.

Meringue

Using a clean bowl and beaters, beat until frothy:

2 egg whites

Add:	**1½ cups brown sugar** **4 tablespoons unsweetened cocoa** **½ teaspoon vanilla** **½ teaspoon almond flavoring**

Continue beating until very stiff. Spread over unbaked base. Bake in 350° oven for 25-30 minutes. Do not overbake. The chocolate meringue should be soft and wet inside.

CHOCOLATE FRUIT SQUARES

Chop very fine and set aside:	**½ cup walnuts** **½ cup mixed fruits**
Beat together:	**¼ cup oil** **2 eggs, less 1 yolk** **¼ cup granulated sugar** **1 cup brown sugar**
Then add:	**4 tablespoons unsweetened cocoa** **¾ cup sifted all-purpose flour** **½ teaspoon baking powder** **1 teaspoon vanilla** **¼ teaspoon salt**
Add:	**fruit and nut mixture**

Bake in a 9 x 9 inch baking pan in 350° oven 15-20 minutes. Do not over-bake, squares should be moist.

Sift: 1 teaspoon confectioners' sugar

through a fine strainer over the squares.

MINCEMEAT SQUARES OR PIE

Filling

Bring to a boil in a saucepan and then set aside:

> 1 box Borden's *Dried* None Such Condensed
>   Mince Meat
> ½ cup raisins
> 2 grated apples
> ¾ cup water

Base

Combine into a dough that resembles coarse meal:

> 1 cup sugar
> ½ cup oil
> ¼ cup skim milk
> 2 cups sifted all-purpose flour
> ⅓ teaspoon baking soda
> ½ teaspoon salt
> 1 teaspoon baking powder

Press ⅔ of the dough firmly into a 9 x 13 inch pan. Spread the filling over the raw dough. Grate the remaining dough over the filling. Bake in a 400° oven for 20-30 minutes. Bake this same recipe in a large pie plate and you will have a delicious, hot mincemeat pie.

DATE SQUARES

Cook, stirring occasionally:

> ½ pound pitted dates
> ½ cup water
> ½ cup sugar
> 1 teaspoon lemon juice

When dates are soft, set aside.

Sift:

> 1 cup sifted all-purpose flour
> ½ teaspoon baking powder
> ¼ teaspoon baking soda
> ½ teaspoon salt

Add:

> 1¼ cups rolled oats (not instant)
> ⅓ cup brown sugar

Blend in with a fork:

> ½ cup oil

Sprinkle half of the rolled oat mixture in lightly oiled 8 x 8 inch pan. Press down with fingers. Spread with date mixture. Sprinkle remaining dough over dates and press down lightly. Bake in 350° oven for 45 minutes or until lightly browned. Cut into squares while still warm.

OATMEAL SNACK BARS

Combine:	1 cup oil
	½ cup brown sugar
	½ cup granulated sugar
Add, beating until well mixed:	2 eggs
	2 teaspoons vanilla
Stir in:	1 cup sifted all-purpose flour
	½ teaspoon salt
	1 cup rolled oats—quick cooking, not instant

Spread batter in a lightly oiled 9 x 13 inch pan. Bake in a 350° oven for 20 minutes. When squares have cooled, glaze with a thin layer of your favorite "chocolate" icing. Cut into bars for serving.

SOUTHERN PECAN BARS

Beat together:	¼ cup oil
	⅓ cup firmly packed brown sugar
	¼ teaspoon salt
Add:	1 cup sifted all-purpose flour
	¼ teaspoon baking powder

Beat until mixture resembles coarse meal. Pat firmly into 9-inch square pan. Bake in 350° oven for 10 minutes.

To make topping, beat until foamy:

2 eggs

Add:	¾ cup dark corn syrup
	¼ cup firmly packed brown sugar
	¼ teaspoon salt
	1 teaspoon vanilla
	2 tablespoons flour

Pour over partially baked crust, then arrange:

1 cup pecan halves on top

Bake in 350° oven 20-25 minutes longer. Let cool and cut into bars.

PANUCHE SQUARES

Beat until light and fluffy:	½ cup oil
	¼ cup granulated sugar
	½ cup firmly packed brown sugar

Then add, mixing thoroughly:	2 egg yolks 2 tablespoons cold water 1 teaspoon vanilla ¼ cup skim milk powder
Sift together and then add:	2 cups sifted all-purpose flour 1 teaspoon baking powder ½ teaspoon salt ⅛ teaspoon baking soda

Spread in a lightly oiled 9 x 13 inch pan.

Beat until frothy:	2 egg whites
Gradually add:	1½ cups firmly packed brown sugar
Spread over cookie dough and sprinkle with:	1 cup chopped walnuts (nuts may be left out, in which case one or two finely grated nuts may be sprinkled over meringue)

Bake in a slow 325° oven for 25-30 minutes. Cut into squares or bars while still warm.

CHOCOLATE PINEAPPLE SQUARES

Combine:	1 cup sugar ⅓ cup unsweetened cocoa 2 cups sifted all-purpose flour ¼ teaspoon salt
Add and mix thoroughly:	1 cup oil 1 egg 2 teaspoons vanilla

Reserve 4 tablespoons of dough and pat the remainder into a 9 x 13 inch baking pan.

Prepare filling by mixing together:

1 can crushed pineapple (20 ounces, not drained)
⅔ cup sugar
2 eggs, less 1 yolk
¼ cup all-purpose flour

Pour filling on top of the dough. Grate the reserved dough over the pineapple mixture using a coarse shredder (or crumble with fingers). Bake in a 350° oven for 40-45 minutes or until filling has set. Cut into squares or diamond shapes when cool.

DATE AND NUT BARS

Combine:	¼ cup oil ¾ cup sugar

                    2 eggs
                    ⅛ teaspoon salt

Sift together   **¾ cup sifted all-purpose flour**
and then add: **¼ teaspoon baking powder**
                    1 cup dates, cut finely
                    ½ cup chopped walnuts
                    rind of an orange, grated

Spread in a lightly oiled 9 x 9 inch pan. Bake in 350° oven for 20-25 minutes. Cut into squares when cool. Raisins may be substituted for the dates if desired.

BLENDER CHEESE SQUARES

These squares can also be made with an electric mixer, but sieve the cheese first and then beat at high speed. Prepare an 8 x 8 inch baking pan by lightly oiling and then sprinkling with a thin layer of:

                    graham cracker crumbs

Blend until smooth: **1½ pounds cottage cheese**
                    2 eggs
                    ½ cup sugar
                    ⅛ teaspoon salt

Remove cheese mixture from blender and stir in:

                    ¾ cup well-drained, crushed pineapple
                    ½ teaspoon lemon rind

Pour cheese mixture into prepared pan and cover with a mixture of:

                    3 tablespoons graham cracker crumbs
                    1 tablespoon sugar
                    ¼ teaspoon cinnamon
                    1 teaspoon oil

Bake in 325° oven for 35 minutes. Cool, then refrigerate.

MARBLE SQUARES (MARSHMALLOW SQUARES)

Beat: **2 tablespoons oil**
                    3 eggs, less 1 yolk
                    ¾ teaspoon vanilla

Add, beating well: **1½ cups brown sugar**
                    ⅓ cup granulated sugar

Then sift together   **1¼ cups sifted all-purpose flour**
and add: **1½ teaspoons baking powder**
                    ½ teaspoon salt

Beat until smooth. Spread half the batter in a lightly oiled 9 x 13 inch pan. To the remaining batter, add:

> **3 tablespoons unsweetened cocoa**
> **¼ cup oil**
> **⅓ cup chopped walnuts**

Drop chocolate mixture evenly by the spoonful onto the white mixture. Marble slightly. Bake in a 350° oven for 20 minutes. Remove from oven and cover with:

> **24 marshmallows**

that have been cut in half (cut side down). Return this to the oven for 2 minutes. Cool to lukewarm and then spread with Rich Cooked Chocolate Icing. Refrigerate for about an hour to facilitate cutting.

Rich Cooked Chocolate Icing

In the top part of a double boiler mix together at low speed of electric mixer:

> **¼ cup oil**
> **⅓ cup unsweetened cocoa**
> **1 egg**
> **½ teaspoon vanilla**
> **1½ cups confectioners' sugar**

Place over simmering water and beat at higher speed until mixture thickens, about 3-5 minutes. If icing is too thick, add a little water a few drops at a time.

DESSERTS AND PIES

FAST UNBAKED PIE SHELL

An unbaked shell can be made by lining a pie plate with a small amount of crushed vanilla wafers, graham cracker crumbs, very thin slices of cake, or chocolate icebox wafers.

PASTRY FOR A TWO-CRUST PIE

In a bowl combine: **2 cups sifted all-purpose flour**
                     1½ teaspoons salt

Pour the following into a bowl but do not stir:

> **⅓ cup cold skim milk ***
> **½ cup oil**

---

* You can use ice water instead of milk. When you do, beat the water with the salad oil blending well, and proceed as above.

Add the liquids to the flour all at once and stir lightly until well mixed. Press the dough into two smooth balls. Wipe the table with a damp cloth (so paper won't slip). Place half of the pastry flattened slightly between 2 12-inch square sheets of waxed paper. Roll out gently until pastry circle reaches edges of paper. If the pastry tears, mend by pressing edges together. Peel off top sheet of paper. Lift bottom sheet of paper and pastry by far corners. Place with paper side up in 8- or 9-inch pie plate. Ease and fit pastry onto plate, gently pull away paper.

Roll top crust in the same way. Lay it over the filling and then cut 3 or 4 small slits in the top. Trim ½ inch beyond pan edge, fold edges under, seal, and flute. Bake as directed. Prepare pastry just before baking. Do not store unbaked.

PASTRY FOR TART SHELLS

Sift together:
- **2 cups sifted all-purpose flour**
- **2 teaspoons sugar**
- **1 teaspoon salt**

Combine in a measuring cup and beat until creamy:
- **⅔ cup oil**
- **4 tablespoons cold skim milk**

Pour liquid all at once into center of flour mixture. Mix until flour is completely dampened. Divide pastry into 24 small or 12 large tart pans. Push evenly with fingers to line bottoms and sides of pans, pressing dough to uniform thickness.

Baked Shells

Prick surface of pastry. Bake in 425° oven about 12 minutes or until browned. Cool in pans. Remove the shells before filling by placing rack over pans and turning over.

Unbaked Shells

Fill with desired filling. Bake tarts according to recipe used. Cool 10 minutes in pan. Prepare pastry just before baking. Do not store unbaked.

NO-ROLL SINGLE SHELL

Sift together in pie plate:
- **1½ cups sifted all-purpose flour**
- **1½ teaspoons sugar**
- **¾ teaspoon salt**

Beat until creamy:
- **½ cup oil**
- **3 tablespoons cold skim milk**

Pour the liquids all at once over the flour. Mix with fork until flour is completely dampened. Push evenly with fingers to uniform thickness lining bottom and sides of pan. To flute, pinch lightly with fingers.

Baked Shell

Prick surface of pastry. Bake in 450° oven for about 12 minutes.

Unbaked Shell

Fill with desired filling and bake according to recipe used. Prepare pastry just before baking. Do not store unbaked.

MERINGUE SHELLS OR TARTS

When making meringue it is very important to have your egg whites at room temperature.

Beat to soft peaks:	**2 egg whites** **¼ teaspoon cream of tartar**
Gradually add:	**½ cup sugar**

Beat until stiff peaks form and sugar is dissolved. Cover a baking sheet with brown paper. Draw 4 circles on the paper, each about 4 inches in diameter (or one 8-inch circle or square). Spread each with meringue, shaping shells with back of spoon. Bake in 275° oven for 1 hour. Turn off heat; let shells dry in oven with door closed for 1 to 2 hours. Set aside until ready to fill.

MANDARIN FILLING FOR MERINGUES

Drain:	**2 11-ounce cans mandarin orange sections**
reserving:	**½ cup of the syrup**
Combine in a saucepan:	**1 tablespoon sugar** **1½ teaspoons cornstarch**

Stir in the reserved syrup. Cook and stir until thickened.

To this syrup add:	**1 tablespoon lemon juice** **¼ teaspoon ground ginger** **drained orange sections**

Chill. Just before serving, spoon the orange mixture into the meringue shells. Fills four shells.

FRESH-FRESH BERRY PIE

Prepare and bake:	**1 9- or 10-inch no-roll pie shell (see recipe in this chapter)**
Blend together:	**¾ cup sugar** **3 tablespoons cornstarch**

1 cup water
2 tablespoons lemon juice

Wash and hull: **3 cups fresh berries**

Crush ⅓ of the berries, reserving the balance. Add crushed berries to the cornstarch mixture. Cook over low heat stirring constantly until thick and clear. Blend with the reserved raw berries and pour into the baked pie shell. Garnish with a few choice berries.

This recipe gives a true berry flavor since only ⅓ of the berries are cooked at all. The rest are still raw.

FRESH APPLE PIE

Prepare pastry for a two-crust pie. Line a 9-inch pie plate with pastry.

Prepare: **6-7 cups thinly sliced tart apples (about 2 pounds)**

Combine: **1-2 teaspoons lemon juice**
½ teaspoon grated lemon rind
1-2 tablespoons flour (if fruit is very juicy)
⅓ cup granulated sugar
⅓ cup brown sugar
¼ teaspoon nutmeg
½ teaspoon cinnamon
⅛ teaspoon salt

Place half of the apples on the unbaked pastry. Sprinkle with half the sugar mixture. Top with the rest of the apples, then sprinkle with the remaining sugar mixture. Place top crust over the fruit, cut slits in the top crust. Sprinkle with a little granulated sugar. Bake in a 400° oven for 40-60 minutes.

FRESH BERRY OR FRUIT PIE

Make and bake as Fresh Apple Pie.

For filling: **4 cups of fruit**

Sugar mixture: **⅔ cup granulated sugar**
2 tablespoons flour
1½ teaspoons lemon juice
¼ teaspoon nutmeg
⅛ teaspoon salt
½ teaspoon grated lemon rind
½ teaspoon cinnamon

CANNED FRUIT PIE

Prepare pastry for a two-crust pie.

Drain: **3 cups canned fruit**

reserving ½ cup juice.

Combine:
   ⅓ cup sugar
   3 tablespoons flour
   ½ teaspoon nutmeg
   ⅛ teaspoon salt
   ½ teaspoon grated lemon rind
   ½ teaspoon cinnamon

Place half of the fruit on the unbaked pastry. Sprinkle with half the sugar mixture. Top with the rest of the fruit, then sprinkle with the remaining sugar mixture.

Pour:
   reserved juice

over the fruit. Place top crust over the fruit, and cut slits in the top crust. Sprinkle with a little:

   sugar

Bake in a 400° oven for 40-60 minutes.

GLAZED FRUIT CREAM PIE

Prepare and bake: 1 9-inch no-roll pie shell

Then prepare according to directions on package:

   1 3-ounce package vanilla pudding (cooked type)

using only: 1¾ cups skim milk

Add: ½ teaspoon almond extract

Cool and pour into baked pie shell.

Arrange over
pudding:
   drained canned peach halves
   or
   any canned fruit combination

Dissolve over
boiling water:
   4 tablespoons red currant or any fruit jelly
   1 tablespoon boiling water

Brush glaze over fruit and chill. This is a good way to use up leftover fruit and provide each member of the family with his favorite fruit pie.

ECLAIRS OR CREAM PUFFS

Heat together just
to the boiling
point:
   1 cup water
   ½ cup oil
   pinch of salt

Add all at once: 1 cup sifted all-purpose flour

Continue cooking stirring constantly until the batter leaves the sides of the pan and forms a ball. Remove from the heat and add:

   4 eggs

(one at a time, beating well after each addition).

Beat until the mixture is very shiny. Using two spoons, form mounds and place on an ungreased cookie sheet, allowing 2 inches between. Bake in a 400° oven for 25 minutes. Reduce heat to 350° and bake 10 minutes longer, or until golden brown. Test the puffs by removing one from the oven and if it doesn't collapse, it is thoroughly done. If the centers are slightly soggy, remove the soggy part. This recipe makes about 12 puffs of a size for an individual dessert.

Unfilled puff shells may be prepared in advance and stored in the refrigerator or freezer. If you want to make eclairs, shape the dough into 4-inch by 1-inch strips instead of mounds.

These puff shells can be filled with many different fillings. You can use a custard filling and top with a chocolate sauce or icing, or fill with commercial vanilla pudding and top with fresh berries. We also fill them with our own ice cream (see recipe in this chapter) and then freeze them for future use. Once the shells are filled with a custard or pudding they must be refrigerated.

BOUCHÉES OR MINIATURE PUFFS

If they are to be used as cases for hors d'oeuvres or small pastries, make them very tiny. Use the recipe above and shape into 1-inch mounds. Bake in 375° oven for 25 minutes. Fill as desired. Unfilled puff shells may be prepared in advance and frozen.

FRENCH-CANADIAN SUGAR TARTS

Prepare:	**1 recipe of tart shells**
Soak:	**¾ cup raisins**

in boiling water for a few minutes until raisins are plump.

Beat until foamy:	**2 tablespoons oil**
	1 egg
	1 cup brown sugar
Add:	**the raisins (drained)**
	1 teaspoon vanilla (or a few teaspoons rum)

Spoon the filling into the uncooked tart shells and bake in a 375° oven for 20 minutes.

NESSELRODE PIE

Bake and set aside:	**1 9-inch pie shell**
In top of double boiler mix together:	**¼ cup skim milk powder**
	1 envelope unflavored gelatin
	¼ cup sugar
	pinch salt

Blend together: **2 egg yolks**
                        1 cup water

Add slowly to gelatin mixture. Cook over hot water stirring constantly until the custard coats a metal spoon and gelatin is dissolved. Remove from heat.

Add: **1 teaspoon rum flavoring**

Chill until mixture begins to thicken to consistency of unbeaten egg whites.

Beat until foamy: **2 egg whites**

Add slowly: **¼ cup sugar**

Beat until stiff peaks form. Fold into the cooled custard.

Add: **¼ cup finely chopped candied fruit**

Pour into baked pie shell. Garnish with finely crushed chocolate icebox wafer crumbs. Refrigerate for a few hours before serving.

SOUTHERN PECAN PIE

Prepare: **1 unbaked 9-inch pie shell**

Combine: **1 cup corn syrup**
                        2 eggs, slightly beaten
                        1 teaspoon vanilla
                        2 tablespoons oil
                        ⅛ teaspoon salt
                        1 cup sugar

Add: **1 cup pecan halves or pieces**

Pour this mixture into the unbaked pie shell. Bake at 400° for 15 minutes, then at 350° for 30 minutes. This pie is done when a knife inserted in the center comes out clean. You can also make this pie with walnuts for a different taste treat.

LEMON MERINGUE PIE

Prepare and bake: **1 9-inch pie shell**

Combine in a   **1 cup sugar**
saucepan: **¼ teaspoon salt**
                        ¼ cup flour
                        3 tablespoons cornstarch

Gradually stir in: **2 cups water**

Cook, stirring constantly, until mixture is thickened and smooth. Gradually stir hot mixture into:

                        2 beaten egg yolks

Return to low heat, and cook stirring two minutes.

Stir in: **¼ cup lemon juice**
                        grated rind of one lemon
                        a few drops of yellow food coloring

Pour into: **baked 9-inch pie shell**

and cool before adding the meringue.

Meringue

This is a meringue for an 8- or 9-inch pie crust.

Beat until frothy: **3 egg whites**

Add: **¼ teaspoon cream of tartar**

and continue beating until the whites are stiff enough to hold a peak.

Gradually beat in: **6 tablespoons of sugar**

and beat until the meringue is stiff and glossy. Spread the meringue lightly on the cooled pie filling until it touches the edges of the pastry. This will prevent the meringue from shrinking. Bake in 400° oven for 5-6 minutes.

When making a lemon meringue pie, you can use one of the commercial pie fillings, but do check the ingredients on the package. We have found coconut oil in many of the ones we have checked, and this is not acceptable.

CREAMY APPLE PUDDING PIE

Prepare and set aside:

                        1 10-inch pie shell, unbaked

Combine: **8 ounces of apple or vanilla skim milk yogurt or**
                          1 cup "sour cream" (see recipe)
                        ⅔ cup sugar
                        1 egg, well beaten
                        ¾ teaspoon vanilla
                        2 tablespoons flour
                        ⅛ teaspoon salt

Beat until smooth.

Stir in: **1 can apple pie filling (1 pound 5 ounces)**

Pour mixture into unbaked pie shell. Bake at 450° for 15 minutes, and then at 325° for 30 minutes. Remove from oven, sprinkle topping over pie, and then continue baking 15 minutes longer.

Topping

Combine: **⅓ cup flour**
                        ¼ cup brown sugar

                    1 teaspoon cinnamon
                    1 tablespoon oil

You can combine other flavors of yogurt and pie filling:

                    Raspberry yogurt with peach pie filling
                    Vanilla yogurt with cherry pie filling
                    Pineapple yogurt with blueberry pie filling

PEACH OR APPLE CRISP

Arrange in a lightly oiled 9 x 12 inch baking dish:

                    15-20 peeled and sliced fresh peaches or apples

Sprinkle them with: **3 teaspoons lemon juice**

Combine until   **1 cup flour**
mixture resembles   **⅛ teaspoon salt**
corn meal: **1¼ cups brown sugar**
                     2½ tablespoons oil
                     1 teaspoon cinnamon

Sprinkle over fruit and bake in 350° oven until fruit is tender and top brown (30-45 minutes).

PEACH FOAM PIE

Prepare and set
aside: **1 9-inch crumb crust**

Beat until lemon colored in top of double boiler (but not over the hot water):

                    2 egg yolks

Add: **¼ cup sugar**
                     ½ teaspoon salt
                     ½ cup skim milk

Now place over boiling water, stirring constantly until the custard coats a spoon. Remove from heat.

Stir in, until   **1 envelope unflavored gelatin soaked in**
well dissolved: **⅓ cup cold water**

Add: **¼ teaspoon almond extract**

Cool.

Combine, and fold   **1 cup frozen or canned peaches, well drained and**
into gelatin   **mashed**
mixture: **1 tablespoon lemon juice**
                     1 teaspoon lemon rind

Beat until frothy: **3 egg whites**

Gradually beat in, and continue beating until stiff:

¼ cup sugar

Gently fold into custard mixture and pour into 9-inch crumb crust. Chill until firm. Garnish with cherries and pistachio nuts.

BLACK BOTTOM PIE

Beat in top of double boiler until light (but not over the hot water):

3 egg yolks

Mix together and then add to egg yolks:
½ cup brown sugar
1½ tablespoons cornstarch
⅛ teaspoon salt

Gradually stir in: **1¾ cups hot skim milk**

Place over hot water. Cook until smooth and thick, stirring constantly, then remove from heat.

Combine:
4 tablespoons cocoa
1 teaspoon vanilla
½ teaspoon almond flavoring
2 tablespoons oil

Gradually add a little of the hot custard until you've added about 1½ cups. Put this chocolate custard in the bottom of a 10-inch pie plate and refrigerate.

To the remaining hot custard add:
1 envelope gelatin softened in
3 tablespoons cold water and
1 teaspoon almond flavoring

For ease in combining, first add some custard to the gelatin until it becomes soft enough to combine. Cool slightly, but do not allow the mixture to set.

Meanwhile beat until frothy:
4 egg whites
¼ teaspoon cream of tartar

Add slowly: **½ cup sugar and beat until stiff**

Fold whites into the slightly cooled custard and pour over the chocolate mixture.

Garnish with: **crushed chocolate wafer crumbs**

Chill until set.

WALDORF PUDDING CAKE

Peel, core, and coarsely chop:

4 medium-sized apples

Add:
- 1 cup sugar
- 1 teaspoon cinnamon
- ½ cup walnuts
- ¾ cup raisins
- ½ teaspoon nutmeg

Set the apple mixture aside.

Sift together:
- 1½ cups sifted all-purpose flour
- 1 teaspoon baking soda
- 1 teaspoon salt

Add, blending well:
- ½ cup oil

Add the batter to the fruit mixture. Mix thoroughly.

Then add:
- 1 beaten egg

Beat for about 2 minutes. Spread into a lightly oiled 8 x 8 inch pan and bake in a 350° oven for 50 minutes. Serve warm with Vanilla Pudding Sauce.

MOCHA FLUFF

In the top of a double boiler combine:
- 1 envelope unflavored gelatin
- 2 tablespoons sugar
- 2 teaspoons instant coffee
- 2 tablespoons unsweetened cocoa
- ¼ teaspoon salt

Beat together:
- 2 egg yolks
- 1½ cups skim milk

Add this gradually to the gelatin mixture and place over hot, not boiling water. Cook stirring constantly until gelatin is dissolved and mixture is slightly thickened. (About 8-10 minutes.) Remove from heat and add:

- 1 teaspoon vanilla

Refrigerate until mixture resembles unbeaten egg whites. Beat until soft peaks form:

- 2 egg whites

Gradually add:
- ¼ cup sugar

and beat until stiff.

Fold into gelatin mixture blending well.

With an electric beater, beat:
- ¼ cup skim milk powder
- ¼ cup ice water
- 1 teaspoon lemon juice

Beat until very stiff (8 minutes) and fold into the gelatin and egg white mixture. Turn into individual dessert dishes or into a 10-inch serving dish. Refrigerate a few hours until set. This is delicious served with Coffee Sauce.

PEACH AND ORANGE MOUSSE

Dissolve: **1 6-ounce package of orange-flavored gelatin**

in: **1 cup hot water and**
                   ½ cup hot peach juice (set the peaches aside)

Cool in refrigerator until the consistency of unbeaten egg whites. Then beat mixture until light and frothy and set aside.

Combine the following and beat until the consistency of whipped cream (8 minutes):

> **¾ cup skim milk powder**
> **¾ cup ice cold water**
> **3 teaspoons lemon juice**

Fold the milk mixture into the gelatin mixture.

Add: **1 cup diced peaches (drained)**

Line a 10-inch pie plate with:

> **¼ cup graham cracker crumbs**

Cover with the peach mixture.

Sprinkle: **2 tablespoons graham cracker crumbs**

over the top and then chill well before serving.

CRÈME D'ORANGE

Sprinkle: **2 envelopes unflavored gelatin over**
                   ½ cup cold water

Add and stir until   **½ cup sugar**
dissolved: **dash of salt**
                     1 cup boiling water

Then add: **1 can (6 ounces) concentrated frozen orange**
                   juice, thawed

Chill until as thick as unbeaten egg whites. Beat the following until the consistency of whipped cream (8 minutes):

> **1 cup skim milk powder**
> **1 cup ice water**
> **4 teaspoons lemon juice**

Gently fold into chilled orange juice mixture. Pour into a 1-quart mold or glass bowl and chill until firm. Unmold just before serving.

Thin: ½ cup orange marmalade with
                             3 tablespoons apricot brandy or orange juice

and serve as a sauce over unmolded crème.

STRAWBERRY CHARLOTTE RUSSE

Combine and stir over low heat until gelatin is dissolved:

> **1 package strawberry gelatin**
> **¼ cup water**
> **¼ cup sugar**

Add: **8-10 marshmallows**

Stir until dissolved and allow to cool. In a large bowl crush:

> **2 cups fresh strawberries**

Add: **¼ cup sugar**
                             2 tablespoons lemon juice
                             2 unbeaten egg whites

Add gelatin mixture to berries, blending well. Chill until slightly thickened. Then whip until thick and light. Whip the following until the consistency of whipped cream (8 minutes):

> **½ cup ice water**
> **½ cup skim milk powder**
> **2 teaspoons lemon juice**

Gently fold whipped milk into beaten berry mixture. Carefully pour into a spring form lined with lady fingers. Refrigerate overnight. Unmold and decorate with large, whole berries. For a particularly festive occasion, serve with thawed frozen strawberries as a sauce.

JELL-O MOUSSE

Dissolve in a saucepan over moderate heat:

> **1 package raspberry gelatin (or any desired flavor)**
> **1¼ cups water**
> **½ cup sugar**

Cool mixture until it just starts to gel. Then whip the following until very thick (8 minutes):

> **½ cup skim milk powder**
> **½ cup ice water**
> **2 teaspoons lemon juice**

Gently fold whipped milk into gelatin mixture. Pour into a spring form that has been lined with lady fingers or a jelly roll sliced very thin. Chill several hours or overnight.

CHOCOLATE MOUSSE

Sprinkle: **1 package unflavored gelatin over**
¼ cup water

Set aside. In a saucepan, blend and cook until smooth, stirring constantly:

3 heaping tablespoons unsweetened cocoa
1 tablespoon oil
¼ cup confectioners' sugar
⅔ cup granulated sugar
¾ cup skim milk

Add the gelatin and stir until well dissolved.

Then add: **1 teaspoon vanilla**
½ teaspoon almond extract

Set saucepan in cold water, stirring occasionally until mixture is thick. Whip the following until thick as whipped cream (about 8 minutes):

⅔ cup skim milk powder
½ cup ice water
1 teaspoon lemon juice

Fold the whipped milk into the chocolate mixture and pour into a 9-inch pie plate lined with chocolate wafers. Chill well.

CROWN JEWELS DESSERT

Prepare and set aside: **½ package each of four bright, strongly colored gelatin flavors (e.g., orange, lime, cherry, wild berry). Use only ¾ cup water for each. Allow each to set in a square, flat pan, about ½-inch deep. Tilt pan slightly to make an uneven layer. When very firmly set, cut into ½-inch squares**

In a saucepan, dissolve thoroughly: **1 package lemon or apple gelatin, using only**
¼ cup sugar
½ cup water

Chill only until the consistency of unbeaten egg whites. Whip the following until very thick (8 minutes):

1 cup skim milk powder
1 cup ice water
4 teaspoons lemon juice

Fold whipped milk into lemon or apple gelatin, then fold colored gelatin pieces into the gelatin-milk mixture. Pour into a large spring form that has been lined with:

chocolate icebox wafers

With a rolling pin or a jar, crush:

2 or 3 chocolate wafers

to a fine powder and sprinkle on top. Chill for several hours before removing from the spring form. Serve on your prettiest serving dish. If you have an oblong serving dish and a long loaf pan, use them, but do not put crumbs on top. Instead, place chocolate biscuits in the bottom of the pan in a pretty pattern and unmold as you would any other mold.

HAPPY AMBROSIA

This should be prepared the night before.

Drain and combine gently:	**1 small can pineapple tidbits (14 ounces)**
	1 can mandarin oranges
	¼ cup maraschino cherries, cut into quarters
	½ cup miniature marshmallows
	2 drops imitation cocoanut extract (optional)
Stir in:	**1 6-ounce container of fruit-flavored skim milk yogurt (we like the peach)**

Chill well overnight. Just before serving, garnish with:

toasted, slivered almonds

You can make this in a much larger quantity for a very pretty party dessert.

MELON DELIGHT

Cut in half:	**6 small cantaloupes**

Scoop out tiny melon balls with a ball cutter. Scallop the cantaloupe shells. Prepare and toss the following with the melon balls:

1 pint raspberries
1 small pineapple, peeled, cored, and diced

Marinate with:	**¼ cup kirsh (or to taste)**

Fill the shells with the fruit and serve cold.

ORANGES IN WINE

In a saucepan, combine:	**1 cup water**
	¾ cup sugar

Stir until the sugar dissolves.

Then add:
> 1 cup red wine (Madeira or any type your family likes)
> 2 cloves
> 1 inch stick cinnamon
> 1 inch vanilla bean
> 4 lemon slices

Bring syrup to a boil and simmer for 15 minutes. Strain, reserving the liquid and set aside.

Peel:
> 6 large oranges

cutting deeply enough to remove outer membrane. Slice thinly. Pour the hot syrup over the slices and refrigerate. Serve chilled.

BAKED APPLES

Although these are called baked apples, they are actually steamed and then broiled—this gives a much nicer apple.

Wash:
> 6 large baking apples

Core the apples without quite cutting through to blossom end. Peel apples about a third of the way down.

In a large covered skillet, combine:
> 2 cups water
> 1 cup sugar
> a few drops of red food coloring
> ½ teaspoon cinnamon

Place apples, peeled side down, in skillet. Cover skillet tightly and steam on top of stove for about 10 minutes. If you don't have a skillet, steam the apples in a large pot and then transfer them to a baking dish for broiling. Carefully turn apples over, re-cover and continue to steam until apples are fork tender—about 15-30 minutes depending on the type of apple used. Watch carefully that you don't overcook. When the apples reach the desired degree of tenderness, sprinkle a bit of sugar over the apples and place them under the broiler for about 10 minutes (not too close to the heat). Constantly baste the apples under the broiler with the syrup so the tops will be well glazed.

BASIC ICE CREAM AND VARIATIONS

Place in top of double boiler:
> 2 tablespoons sugar
> ¼ teaspoon salt
> ⅓ cup skim milk powder made up to ½ cup by adding fruit juice or water
> 8 large marshmallows

Place over boiling water and stir until completely dissolved.

Add:
> 1 teaspoon vanilla

Cool in refrigerator. When cool, whip the following at high speed for 8 minutes until very thick:

> ½ cup skim milk powder
> ½ cup ice water
> 2 teaspoons lemon juice

Fold the milk (whipped) into the marshmallow mixture. When folding 2 mixtures of the same color make sure they are thoroughly mixed because the colors won't guide you. Place at once in flat, rather than deep, covered plastic containers and place in coldest part of freezer. It is a good idea to place a small piece of plastic wrap on the uncovered surface of the ice cream. When the container is not full, the direct surface should always be covered to prevent discoloration and ice crystals.

Variations

1. Canned red pitted cherries cut up make an unbelievably delicious variation—use syrup instead of water and add a few drops of almond extract.
2. Fold in ½ cup fresh strawberries mashed and ½ teaspoon vanilla.
3. Add 2 teaspoons instant coffee dissolved in the marshmallow mixture.
4. Swirl seedless raspberry jam through it.
5. Swirl commercial butterscotch topping through it.
6. Add 2 or 3 drops almond flavoring and ¼ cup toasted, finely sliced almonds.

The combinations are endless. You can make anything Howard Johnson can!

CHOCOLATE ICE CREAM

Combine in top of double boiler, then place over hot water:

> 2 tablespoons unsweetened cocoa (3 if you like it very chocolatey)
> 3 tablespoons sugar
> ⅛ teaspoon salt
> ⅓ cup skim milk powder made up to ½ cup milk with water

Stir until smooth.

Then add:

> 8 large marshmallows

Continue stirring until mixture is smooth. Cool in refrigerator. When marshmallow mixture has cooled, whip the following at high speed for 8 minutes until very thick:

> ½ cup powdered skim milk
> ½ cup ice water
> 2 teaspoons lemon juice

Fold whipped milk into chocolate mixture. Pour at once in flat, rather than deep, covered plastic containers and place in coldest part of freezer.

ICE CREAM CAKE ROLL

Prepare cake roll. Roll in the length and allow to cool. Make chocolate ice cream and freeze in a flat pan. Spread thickly on cake and roll. Wrap well in plastic wrap. Then place in a plastic bag and freeze immediately. This roll can be removed and a few slices taken off at a time. It will keep as long as ice cream will keep.

Serve the chocolate roll with chocolate or marshmallow sauce, or strawberry ice cream with a strawberry sauce. This is a beautiful dessert for company. Place the roll on a platter and sift some confectioners' sugar over the top and have the sauce in your prettiest bowl.

Chapter 20 • Candies, Drinks, Icings and Sauces

This is a special section that you should value very highly. The following recipes clearly separate this program from all others, because these are foods that the dieter is usually required to forego. With our plan for fat-controlled foods, you need not give up any treats. Because of the low-fat content of our recipes, candies, ice cream, and toppings can be enjoyed without worrying about exceeding your fat limit.

In any low-cholesterol plan, for example, chocolate and butter are taboo. This means that all chocolate candies and cream-based candies, fillings, icings, sauces, and syrups have to be omitted unless substitutes can be found. In this book we provide you with the substitutes—not for just candies and sweets, but for all foods that should be avoided. This chapter is the highlight of our process of substitution.

Without these recipes, our plan, too, would have little chance of succeeding because these are the foods that add fun and zest to your eating plan. Any diet can become tiresome if it is confined to basic foods, and if the diet becomes monotonous it will soon be abandoned. That is why every diet, whether low-fat, low-sugar, or low-calorie should have a place for desserts and "treat" types of food. We have provided enough of these to satisfy the sweetest tooth.

Ordering chocolate desserts in restaurants is hazardous, so save these for home consumption. We have recipes for such goodies as chocolate candy, milk shakes, and icing. These can be prepared with the chocolate taste, but without the saturated fat.

Old basics can also be used to provide very fancy desserts. For example, to make a festive sponge or chiffon cake, try our lemon or mocha cream filling instead of whipped cream; or top a plain cake with our strawberry or apricot whip for another variation.

Using these recipes imaginatively will make you proud of leading your family into a whole new mode of eating that provides treats not treatments.

CHOCOLATE FUDGE

Combine in a heavy saucepan and stir constantly over high heat until sugar is dissolved:

> **2 cups sugar**
> **6 tablespoons unsweetened cocoa**
> **¾ cup skim milk**

Then cook very slowly *without* stirring (remove pan from heat for a few seconds if it seems to be cooking too quickly) until soft ball stage—238° (about half an hour). Then remove pan from heat and add without stirring:

> **2 tablespoons oil**

Allow to cool. When nearly cool, add:

> **1 teaspoon vanilla**

Pour into small bowl and beat with electric beater until mixture just starts to thicken (about 5 minutes).

Then add: **1 cup chopped walnuts**

Spread immediately in a lightly oiled 8 x 8 inch pan, and cut into squares while still warm.

PECAN PRALINES

Combine and cook without stirring until it reaches 238° (soft ball stage) on candy thermometer:

> **1 cup granulated sugar**
> **2 cups light brown sugar**
> **¼ cup light corn syrup**
> **⅛ teaspoon salt**
> **1¼ cups skim milk**

Remove from heat and cool to lukewarm.

Then add: **1 teaspoon vanilla**

Add: **1½ cups unbroken pecan halves**

Beat with spoon until mixture thickens and loses its gloss. Drop by spoonfuls onto waxed paper. Let stand until firm. Then wrap in plastic wrap or waxed paper. Store in an air-tight container.

BRANDY COCOA BALLS

Combine: **1 cup finely crushed vanilla wafers**
          1 cup sifted confectioners' sugar
          1 cup chopped pecans
          2 tablespoons unsweetened cocoa
          2 tablespoons light corn syrup

¼ cup brandy (1 teaspoon almond extract and orange juice may be substituted)

Mix well and shape into 1-inch balls. Roll the balls in any of the following:

**finely chopped pecans
dry cocoa
granulated sugar**

Store in refrigerator.

CANDIED ORANGE OR GRAPEFRUIT PEEL

Cut into strips, the peel from:

2 oranges or 1 grapefruit

Cover with cold water and bring slowly to a boil. Drain well and start again with fresh water. Repeat until the peel has been boiled 5 times.

Make a syrup of: **½ cup sugar
¼ cup water**

Add the peel and boil slowly until all syrup is absorbed. Cool the peel, then roll it in:

sugar

Allow to dry and store in a tightly covered box. It will keep indefinitely.

APRICOT-ORANGE CANDY

Wash, pat dry,
and set aside: **25 dried apricot halves, the largest you can find**

Put the following through a meat grinder using the fine blade:

½ cup candied orange peel or mixed peels

Thin to a sticky consistency with:

2-4 teaspoons corn syrup or honey

Spread ½ teaspoonful between apricot halves and stick together in pairs to form sandwiches. Place each in a paper candy cup. These will keep for weeks in the refrigerator.

CHOCOLATE-DIPPED FRUITS AND NUTS

Stir together with a spoon until right consistency for dipping, adding very small amounts of sugar or yogurt to vary the consistency:

**1 cup confectioners' sugar, sifted
3 tablespoons cocoa, sifted
2 tablespoons vanilla skim milk yogurt
1 tablespoon oil**

Prepare for dipping enough fruit and nuts for about 40 candies:

large toasted almonds
large pecans or walnut halves
marshmallows cut into quarters
pitted prunes
dried apricots
glazed fruits
raisins or peanuts

Dip one at a time in the chocolate mixture. Remove with a fork, shake off excess chocolate, and place on a foil-covered cookie sheet. Tweezers may be used to handle the small pieces. When you have used about ¾ of the chocolate mixture, add raisins or peanuts and mix. Keep adding raisins until all are covered. Then drop by the teaspoonful on the cookie sheet. Place in the refrigerator. The candy will harden. Turn raisin or peanut clusters so that the bottom sides can harden. Store in a covered container in the refrigerator. They will keep for weeks.

HEAVENLY HASH OR ROCKY ROAD

Make chocolate covering for Dipped Fruits and Nuts.

Then stir in:　　**30 marshmallows cut in halves (colored if desired)**
　　　　　　　　½ cup coarsely cut toasted almonds or pecans

Pack firmly into foil-lined pan and refrigerate until firm. Cut into squares. Store covered in the refrigerator.

DATE BALLS

Put through meat grinder:
2 cups corn flakes or any other dry cereal
¾ cup pitted dates or prunes
½ cup pecans

To this mixture add:
2 tablespoons honey or corn syrup
1 tablespoon oil
2 teaspoons lemon juice
½ teaspoon lemon rind

Mix well. Shape into small balls and roll in:

powdered fruit sugar

Top with pecan halves.

CINNAMON-SUGARED ALMONDS

Combine in a saucepan:
1¼ cups sugar
½ cup water
1 teaspoon cinnamon
1 pound unblanched almonds

234 / CANDIES, DRINKS, ICINGS AND SAUCES

234 / CANDIES, DRINKS, ICINGS AND SAUCES

Cook over medium heat. Stir occasionally to coat all the nuts. Continue cooking until the liquid is evaporated. Immediately spread the nuts on a cookie sheet and bake in 375° oven for 10 minutes. These nuts keep very well in a covered container and they freeze beautifully.

CREAMY PEPPERMINTS

Stir over low heat until dissolved:

2 cups sugar
¼ cup light corn syrup
¼ cup skim milk
¼ teaspoon cream of tartar

Cook slowly until soft ball stage—238°. Remove from heat, cool slightly. Beat until creamy.

Then add:

8-10 drops of oil of peppermint
or
½ teaspoon spearmint flavoring (or desired flavoring)

Color with vegetable coloring as desired. Drop from teaspoon onto waxed paper to harden. These may then be chocolate dipped.

BLENDER FRUIT SHAKE

In a blender combine:

½ cup fresh or frozen strawberries
⅓ cup skim milk powder
2 tablespoons sugar
1 teaspoon lemon juice
dash of salt

Cover and blend at medium speed until smooth.

Add:

1 cup crushed ice

Blend again for one minute and serve immediately. Any of the following fruits may be combined or substituted:

bananas
fresh or canned peaches
fresh or canned cherries
fresh or canned apricots

or use your own variations.

FROSTED ORANGE DRINK

Combine the following in a blender:

1 cup orange juice
½ cup skim milk powder
½ tablespoon sugar

drop of vanilla extract
½ cup crushed ice

Blend until frothy and serve at once.

MOCHA FROSTED DRINK

Combine in
blender:

1 cup water
1 cup crushed ice
½ cup skim milk powder
4 tablespoons sugar
1 tablespoon cocoa
½ teaspoon instant coffee
2 drops vanilla
a few grains of salt

Blend for half a minute. If only an electric mixer is available, beat at high speed for 2 minutes.

HOT MOCHA COFFEE

Combine, then
divide into 2 cups:

1 teaspoon instant coffee
1 teaspoon cocoa
⅛ teaspoon cinnamon
⅛ teaspoon nutmeg
dash of salt
2½ teaspoons sugar
2 tablespoons skim milk powder

Add enough boiling water and stir to dissolve all granules. Then fill cups with more boiling water and float several miniature marshmallows on top.

COFFEE ICING GLAZE

Beat together:

1 tablespoon oil
1 teaspoon instant coffee dissolved in
1 tablespoon cold water
1 cup confectioners' sugar

Very slowly add enough:

skim milk

to thin to desired consistency for spreading. This will cover a 9 x 13 inch cake.

SOFT CHOCOLATE ICING

Boil together over
low heat, stirring
frequently:

⅓ cup unsweetened cocoa
3 tablespoons cornstarch
1⅓ cups sugar

1½ cups skim milk
2 tablespoons skim milk powder
pinch of salt

When slightly thickened (about 10 minutes after boiling) remove from heat and add:

1 teaspoon vanilla (or ½ teaspoon almond extract)
1 teaspoon oil

Pour over cake. This will thicken to a hot fudge sauce consistency.

CHOCOLATE YOGURT ICING

Blend together with a fork:

1 cup confectioners' sugar
1½ tablespoons unsweetened cocoa
2 tablespoons vanilla-flavored skim milk yogurt

Since each brand of yogurt is of a slightly different consistency, you may have to adjust the amount of yogurt you add. Start with 1½ tablespoons and continue adding until desired consistency.

BASIC CHOCOLATE ICING

Combine and mix thoroughly:

1 tablespoon oil
1½ cups sifted confectioners' sugar
4 tablespoons unsweetened cocoa
3 tablespoons skim milk
½ teaspoon vanilla

Add a little more milk until the icing is of the desired consistency, adding only a few drops at a time.

SEVEN-MINUTE ICING

Combine in top of double boiler:

1 egg white
¾ cup sugar
2½ tablespoons cold water
⅛ teaspoon cream of tartar

Place over boiling water, beating with electric mixer, until peaks form (approximately 7 minutes). Remove from heat.

Add:

½ teaspoon vanilla

Continue beating until proper consistency for spreading. Drizzle or splatter small amounts of chocolate syrup over this icing.

BROWN SUGAR FLUFFY ICING

Combine in top of double boiler:

1 egg white
¾ cup brown sugar

½ teaspoon corn syrup
1 tablespoon cold water

Then place over boiling water and continue beating with electric beater until thick.

Add: 1 teaspoon vanilla

Spread over cake.

MOCHA CREAM FILLING

Combine in a saucepan:	½ cup sugar
	3 tablespoons flour
	2 teaspoons instant coffee
	¼ teaspoon salt
	2 tablespoons cocoa
	1 tablespoon oil
Add:	1¼ cups skim milk

Cook and stir until thickened. Cook 2 minutes longer. Stir small amount of hot mixture into:

1 beaten egg, less half the yolk

Return the mixture to the saucepan. Cook and stir until just boiling.

Then add: 1 teaspoon vanilla

Cool and fiill desired cake.

TART LEMON FILLING

Combine in a saucepan:	1 cup sugar
	2 tablespoons water
	4 tablespoons cornstarch
	¼ teaspoon salt
Stir in gradually:	½ cup orange juice
	½ cup lemon juice
	1 tablespoon oil
Then add:	½ teaspoon grated lemon rind

Bring to a boil over moderate heat, stirring constantly. Boil for 1 minute.

ORANGE FILLING

Combine in a saucepan:	1 cup sugar
	4 tablespoons cornstarch
	¼ teaspoon salt
Stir in gradually:	1 cup orange juice
	2 tablespoons grated orange rind

2 tablespoons lemon juice
1 tablespoon oil

Bring to a boil over moderate heat, stirring constantly. Boil 1 minute. Cool.

STRAWBERRY WHIP

Whip together at high speed:

1 egg white
1¼ cups hulled raw strawberries, well drained
¼ cup sugar

Continue beating until thick as whipped cream.

Add:

2 drops almond extract
or
½ teaspoon lemon juice

Pile into sherbet dishes and refrigerate or serve as a sauce over sliced angel food cake. If there is any left over it will rewhip the next day. This holds its texture for about 2 to 3 hours.

APRICOT WHIP

Beat until stiff:

1 egg white
2 tablespoons sugar

When stiff, add:

¼ cup sieved, cooked dry apricots

Serve in sherbet dishes or as a sauce for a plain cake.

HOT ORANGE SAUCE

Simmer together for 10 or 15 minutes:

1 teaspoon oil
2 tablespoons sugar
2 tablespoons finely grated orange rind
¾ cup orange juice
2 tablespoons lemon juice

Can be prepared in advance—reheat and serve as a sauce.

HOT FUDGE SAUCE

In a saucepan combine:

⅓ cup unsweetened cocoa
1 cup sugar
2 tablespoons flour
2 tablespoons cornstarch
1½ cups water

Cook over medium heat, stirring constantly until mixture comes to a full boil and thickens. Remove from heat and add:

1 teaspoon vanilla

Serve warm.

If you have any sauce left over, it can be stored in the refrigerator. To re-heat, place in a pan over hot (not boiling) water until the sauce is of pouring consistency.

COFFEE SAUCE

Combine in
saucepan:

½ cup sugar
1 tablespoon flour
1 tablespoon cornstarch
1 teaspoon instant coffee
⅛ teaspoon salt
¾ cup water

Cook over medium heat stirring constantly, until clear and slightly thick-ened. Serve hot.

CARAMEL SYRUP

Place in large heavy skillet over medium heat:

2 cups sugar

Allow to cook slowly, stirring constantly until the sugar is liquid and pale golden. Remove from heat and add:

2 cups boiling water

very very *slowly*, so that the steam does not burn you. Return to heat and con-tinue cooking until slightly thickened. This syrup will thicken when it cools. If desired, a few drops of maple extract may be added and you have a very inexpensive maple syrup. Store covered in a jar in refrigerator and it keeps indefinitely.

VANILLA PUDDING SAUCE

Mix thoroughly:

½ cup sugar
dash of salt
1 tablespoon cornstarch

Add:

¼ cup cold water

and stir to a thin paste.

Combine in a
saucepan:

½ cup boiling water
1 tablespoon oil

Add the paste and cook over medium heat, stirring constantly, until mix-ture thickens slightly and comes to a boil.

Cool and add: **1 teaspoon vanilla**

May be stored in a covered jar in the refrigerator for up to one week.

SPEEDY CHOCOLATE SYRUP

Place in saucepan and mix well:	½ cup unsweetened cocoa
	1¼ cups sugar
Add:	1¼ cups boiling water

Stir until smooth. Place over low heat and boil for one minute. Remove from heat.

| Add: | 1 teaspoon vanilla |

Pour into jar and store covered in refrigerator. This syrup is perfect for making chocolate milk.

FRUIT SAUCES

Heat canned blueberry pie filling, adding enough water to make a good sauce consistency and serve over a plain cake. Any fruit filling may be used this way.

"WHIPPED CREAM" TOPPING

| Dissolve: | 1 teaspoon unflavored gelatin in |
| | 1 tablespoon hot water |

You can do this by putting the mixture in a small glass over hot water and stirring until dissolved. Then set aside.

Beat until very stiff (8 minutes):	½ cup ice water
	½ cup skim milk powder
	1 tablespoon lemon juice
	1 teaspoon vanilla
When stiff, add very *slowly*:	⅓ cup sugar
	the dissolved gelatin

Pour into a plastic container and store in the freezer. Remove by the spoonful as desired. Will keep 4-6 weeks.

Glossary

Cholesterol
A waxy material used in many of the body's chemical processes. Everyone requires it in correct amounts, but too much in the circulatory system encourages the development of heart disease. It is manufactured by the body from fats, or can be obtained directly from foods of animal origin.

Fat
A chemical substance that can be solid or liquid, depending on the type. Solid fat is usually saturated, and liquid fat is usually unsaturated.

"Low-fat"
This label on a food product is not meaningful for our purposes, and can be misleading. The question is, how low is the fat content and how much of the fat is saturated.

Marbling in Meat
Fat that is distributed throughout the meat and cannot be removed, as in steaks and roasts. It is barely visible as small, white lines running through raw meat, producing a marbleized appearance.

Monounsaturated Fats
These are neutral fats that have little or no effect on the level of cholesterol in the blood. Olive oil is one example of a monounsaturated fat.

Oil
A type of fat that is liquid at room temperature.

Polyunsaturated Fats
The healthiest form of unsaturated fats.

Saturated Animal Fats
Fats found in beef, lamb, pork, and whole-milk products, such as butter, cream, and cheese.

Saturated Fats
Fats, usually solid at room temperature, that are harmful when consumed beyond certain limits. They are found in most animal products and in some hydrogenated vegetable products. The word "saturated" refers to a characteristic of their chemical activity.

Saturated Vegetable Fats
Fats found in many solid or hydrogenated shortenings and in coconut oil, cocoa butter, and palm oil. Palm oil and coconut oil are used in many commercially prepared cookies, pie fillings, and most nondairy milk and cream substitutes.

Separable Fat
Fat that can be easily removed from a piece of raw meat.

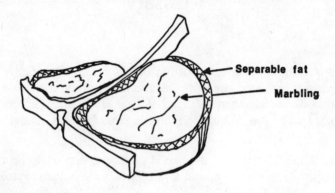

Special Margarine
A type of partially hardened margarine prepared from vegetable oils. These margarines are less harmful than ordinary margarines because they contain less saturated fat. Special margarines list "liquid oil" as the first and therefore primary ingredient.

Unsaturated Fats
Usually these fats are liquid oils of vegetable origin. Oils from corn, cottonseed, safflower, sesame seed, soybeans, and sunflower seed are high in unsaturated fat. They are considered beneficial to health because they tend to lower the level of cholesterol in the blood.

General Index

Recipe Index

Bibliography

Bierenbaum, M. L. et al., Modified-fat dietary management of the young male with coronary disease, JAMA, 202:1119–1123, December, 1967

Dayton, S. et al., Prevention of coronary heart disease and other complications of arteriosclerosis by modified diet, Am. J. of Med., 46:751–762, May, 1969

Ford, C. M. et al., An institutional approach to the dietary regulation of blood cholesterol in adolescent males, Prev. Med., 1:426–445, 1972

Turpeinen, O. et al., Blood lipids and primary coronary events: the effects of diet modification, Minn. Med., 52:1247–1252, August, 1969